CANCELLED

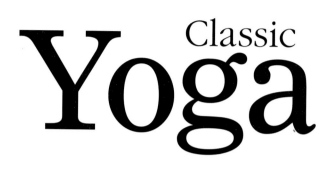

Classic Yoga

Vimla Lalvani

Classic
Yoga

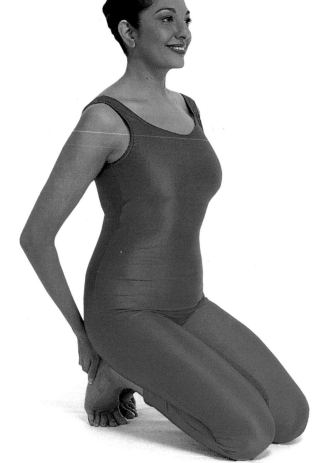

Vimla Lalvani

CHANCELLOR
PRESS

Course One 23

Course Two 51

Contents

First published in hardback in Great Britain in 1996
by Hamlyn

This edition published 2002 by Chancellor Press,
an imprint of Bounty Books, a division of
Octopus Publishing Group Ltd,
2-4 Heron Quays, London E14 4JP
Text © The Natural Therapy Company Limited 1998

Design © Octopus Publishing Group Limited 1996

Photographs © Octopus Publishing Group Limited 1996

NOTE
It is advisable to check with your doctor before embarking on any exercise
program. Yoga should not be considered a replacement for professional medical
treatment; a physician should be consulted in all matters relating to health and
particularly in respect of pregnancy and any symptoms which may require

ISBN 0 7537 0627 X

A CIP catalogue record for this book is available from the British Library.

Printed in China by Toppan Printing Co., (H.K.) Ltd.

diagnosis or medical attention. While the advice and information in this book
are believed to be accurate and the step-by-step instructions have been devised to
avoid strain, neither the author nor the publisher can accept any legal
responsibility for any injury sustained while following the exercises.

Introduction

What is Yoga?

Many people want to know what yoga is and how it can help them. In this book I hope to explain classical yoga in a modern sense and to de-mystify the principles of yoga philosophy. The benefits of yoga are many and people who practice regularly will see a great change in their physical body and their whole mental outlook.

Given the stresses and strains of our daily lives, we must learn the art of shutting ourselves away from

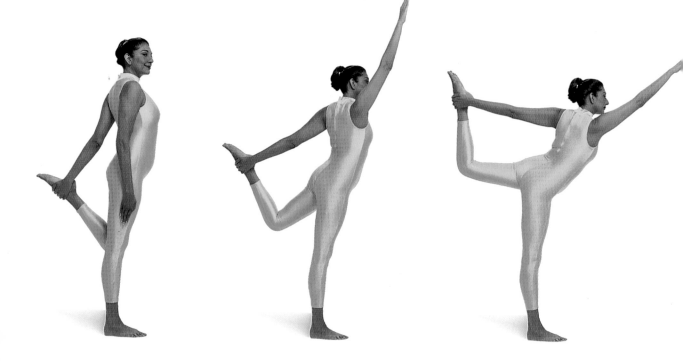

chaos and retreating into our inner selves to find peace, balance and harmony. Yoga teaches you how to achieve this. *Classic Yoga* explains how yoga can improve your everyday life. You will discover the real you and experience 'yoga living'. You will learn the techniques of yoga and understand the mental and physical aspects of the philosophy.

In Sanskrit, the word 'yoga' means the union of mind and body. Yoga is not a religion but a philosophy of life. It is an ancient science of movement developed in India thousands of years ago to improve all aspects of your life, both mental and physical. The main principle of yoga is that mastery over the mind and senses will lead to a cessation of misery and bring you salvation.

The Paths of Yoga

There are five different forms of yoga and for maximum benefit they should be practiced together. The four mental yogas are Bhakti yoga (emotions), Gyana yoga (wisdom), Raja yoga (meditation) and Karma yoga (actions). The one physical yoga is called Hatha yoga. In

'masculine' or 'feminine' are largely shared by men and women, it is essential that both energies are balanced equally. Yoga is the art and science of balance in everyday living and moderation in all that we do. It teaches us how to have harmonious relationships with others and how to understand our own inner truth. It connects us to our souls and sets us on a path of true spirituality. The ultimate goal for the yogi is to join the spiritual self to the cosmic energy of the universe.

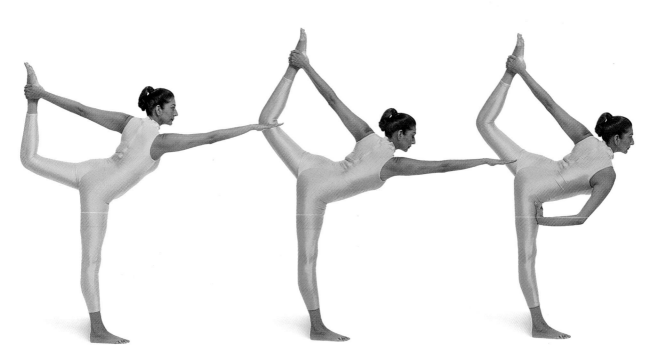

this book we concentrate on Hatha yoga because it is the first stage of development; yoga philosophy states that before you can have a disciplined mind you must first begin to train your body.

Hatha yoga is a series of asanas, or postures, that train and discipline the body and mind. In Sanskrit, 'ha' means the sun or male energy and 'tha' the moon or female energy. When you practice the asanas you are combining and balancing the masculine and feminine energies which are within all of us, whether male or female. In the Western world today, where professions, tasks and hobbies that were once considered exclusively

Hatha Yoga

Hatha yoga exercises the glands, organs and nerves in the body as well as toning the muscles. The yoga exercises are divided between asanas (exercise positions), Pranayama (breath control), Raj asanas (meditative postures), and Nauli, Mudras and Bandhas (purifying and cleansing postures). The exercises might appear strange when you first begin but as you familiarize yourself with the sequences you will understand how they work. Fluid movements unblock energy and, combined with correct breathing, increase your vitality and discipline your mind.

Yoga for Today

The popularity of yoga has soared in recent years. Attitudes to health, spirituality, lifestyle and mankind's place in the environment have changed dramatically and people are seeking solutions to the problems of their everyday existence. In these confusing times, the environment is struggling for survival and we are suffering from mental and physical stress, with some new diseases making an appearance and old ones thought to have been conquered by antibiotics reasserting themselves. We cannot always change these

The Physical Benefits of Yoga

Yoga is totally different from other types of exercise. First of all, it is non-competitive. The purpose of yoga is to understand yourself through your yoga practice and to work slowly and deliberately to gain flexibility as you progress. It is the antithesis of the 'no pain, no gain' philosophy. Graceful, fluid movements replace pounding flesh, creating a balance and strength of the mind, body and spirit.

The purpose is not to build muscle but to build muscle tone. In yoga asanas the muscles are stretched

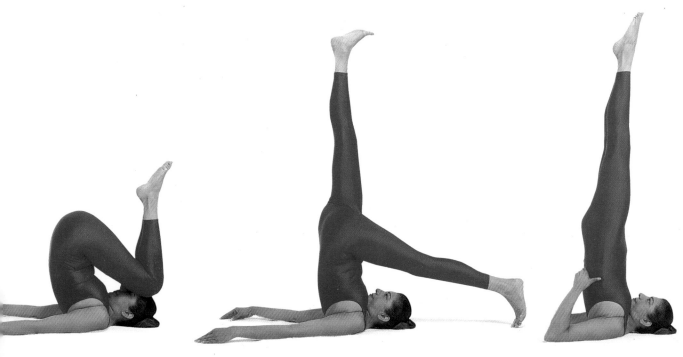

conditions but we can learn to cope with them. Yoga provides a perfect solution because it brings harmony and balance to your life; because your mental state is balanced you will be able to solve problems calmly and rationally, and because your physical health is improved you will have a better resistance to illnesses.

The yoga system is based on universal truths, so it does not interfere with anyone's religious beliefs. Yoga is for men and women of all ages and occupations and you can begin to learn at any time. Everyone's life is transformed and enriched by a new outlook, improved health, a new awareness and a fresh philosophy.

lengthwise. Fat is eliminated around the cells and, combined with correct breathing, the exercises will improve the circulation and release toxin build-up. This process will reduce cellulite.

Yoga asanas also regulate the metabolism which controls weight gain and loss. As we grow older the metabolism slows down automatically. Continued practice of yoga postures keeps the metabolism rate stable so your weight will not fluctuate, and you will be able to maintain your ideal weight. Yoga also builds the immune system, so you will rarely experience even a common cold, and exercises the internal organs so that the body will work like a finely tuned car which runs in peak condition.

Yoga also helps to ease physical tensions through deep stretching and correct breathing techniques. Working on the physical body with deep concentration on breathing creates a real and lasting sense of harmony, embracing the body and mind. Yoga is a wonderful way of learning how to relax. The physical techniques create a calm and concentration that extend beyond the body deep into the mind, effectively reducing stress at all levels.

Many people are quite content to continue with Hatha yoga and benefit from the new-found discipline. Others discover a need to go further. Yoga opens the mind to a certain stillness and clarity and many people find they wish to pursue a spiritual path. Yoga raises the conscious level and brings the soul, mind and body into union by means of eight disciplines: Yama (ethics); Niyama (religious observances); Asana (postures); Pranayama (breathing exercises) Pratyahara (withdrawal of senses from objects); Dharana (concentration); Dhyana (meditation); Samadhi (superconsciousness).

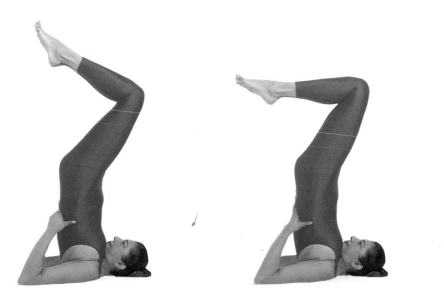

Diet and Lifestyle

Many people believe that in order to begin studying yoga they must change their habits. They may well fear that they will be told to give up meat, alcohol and smoking overnight! In fact, yoga is not about abstinence at all – rather, it is about the art of moderation.

In yoga, there are no fixed rules laid down about what is permissible. However, because the philosophy is about returning your body to its natural equilibrium you will not feel the need for excesses. When your mind and body are in harmony and you are in tune with yourself you will want to maintain a healthy, balanced lifestyle.

The Chakras

In the Sanskrit language, the word 'chakra' means 'wheel'. Chakras are 'wheels' that radiate energy in a circular motion through the vital centres of the spine. Just as antennae are able to pick up radio waves and transform them into sound, so chakras pick up cosmic vibrations and distribute them throughout the body via these energy centers.

In the spine we have seven chakras or energy centers moving from the tail bone up to the top of the head. Each center controls different senses, and all these centers must flow freely to maintain good health.

Many people have blocked chakras, and yoga exercises unblock them. The twisting and turning of the body stretches the nerves and the increased supply of oxygen cleanses and purifies the bloodstream. Every cell is renewed and the energy flows smoothly.

I like to use a hosepipe as an analogy. When there is a kink in the pipe the water will trickle out slowly and unevenly; when the pipe is unkinked the water will flow strongly. It is exactly the same in the case of energy. When the chakras are unblocked the energy flow will be powerful and dynamic.

Clasp your hands over your head and continue to stretch your arms up while keeping your knees and shoulders down. Feel your fingertips tingling with energy and release your hands in a sudden burst. You will be surprised at how energized and powerful you feel as a result of carrying out this simple exercise.

All yogic exercises are based on a formula of stretching, relaxation and deep breathing to increase the circulation and improve concentration. In the meditative poses, sitting while breathing deeply reduces the metabolic rate. When the body is kept in this steady

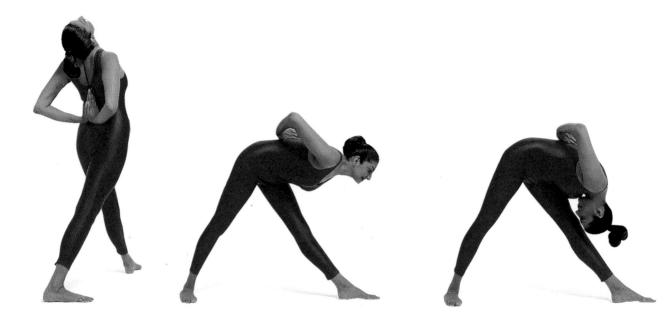

It is important for you to be able to visualize the energy moving through your spine and there is a technique that will allow you to experience this. Sit upright on the floor, preferably in a cross-legged or lotus position. Look over your surroundings, close your eyes and relax the muscles of your face. Begin to breathe deeply and slowly. Become aware of the energy in the base of your spine. Feel bliss, calm and serenity. Stretch your arms out to the sides of your body with your palms facing upward. Gradually raise your arms and visualize the energy slowly moving to the center of your spine, then between the shoulder blades, up through the base of your neck and on through to the very top of your head.

pose for some time, the mind becomes free of physiological disturbances caused by physical activity. There is a steady flow of nerve energy that electrifies the body and awakens the spiritual power in man through breathing techniques and concentration. The Raj asanas prepare you for meditation – focusing your mind on one thought. It is a scientific approach that you can apply to many areas of your life. When you rid your mind of useless thoughts, clarity is increased and you can find your own solutions rather than relying on a third party. This is one of the goals of the aspiring yogi. You will experience the power and joy of yoga when you can master your own thoughts and actions.

How to Use This Book

For this book I have specifically designed three yoga courses which are based on different levels of fitness and experience of yoga. The main objective of the book is to teach you the basics of yoga and to guide your progress through to Course 3. Before you begin Course 1, it is important that you become familiar with the safety guidelines (page 12), breath control (page 13) and correct posture (page 14). Before embarking on any course you should follow the warm-up (page 16) and cool down afterward with a relaxation routine (page 22).

suppleness. As you move into the more challenging yoga asanas you will feel a sense of elation in your ability to tackle these difficult poses; you will become energized and motivated, yet your mood will be calm.

The real challenge begins in Course 3, because the exercises combine the need for balance along with physical strength and stamina. They will show you immediately what your mental state is – some days you will be surprised by your skill and other days you will need a sense of humor! As you are different every day, so your yoga practice will be too; the most important

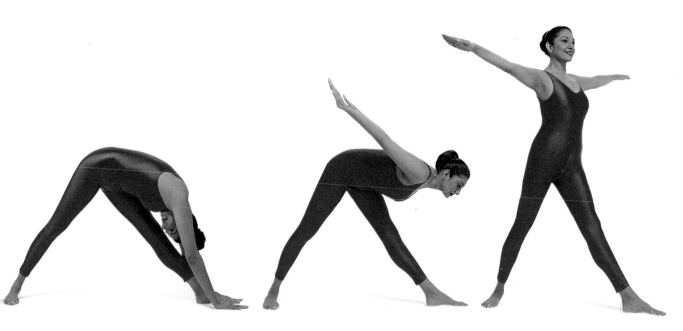

Course 1 is a foundation course in which you will learn the importance of breathing correctly and of aligning the spine. The yoga exercises are very gentle, slow and easy to follow, and will teach you to move in a new way. These exercises are linked with a specific breathing pattern which will allow your energy to alter and flow freely through the system. Keep your mind focused on what your body is doing as you are practicing them and try to maintain a calm frame of mind.

When you are sure you have thoroughly mastered Course 1 you can then move on to Course 2. This course presents you with more dynamic exercises which, you will quickly discover, call for more strength, stamina and

aspect to bear in mind is never to become discouraged.

You will probably find that you are able to do some asanas better on one side than the other. This is because our natural energy differs and some people are happier doing grounding exercises while others like to fly. The rule here is to try to do each asana equally well and to concentrate especially on those that you find difficult. In fact, when you experience difficulty it means that the area is weak and requires balancing. Yoga is a discipline, so only continued practice will show results. The results will be dynamic: an invigorated body, increased stamina, improved muscle tone and a feeling of total harmony and calm.

Explanation of Terms Used in This Book

◆ For first position, stand tall in perfect posture with your feet together.

◆ For second position, stand tall in perfect posture with your feet apart, directly under the hip bones, and toes pointing forward. If an exercise calls for wide second position, place your feet 1–1.2m (3–4ft) apart.

◆ To center yourself, concentrate on the solar plexus while breathing deeply. This helps to balance your physical and mental state.

◆ To lift your spine, concentrate on the tail bone (the coccyx) while lifting your spine straight.

◆ To open the chest, push your shoulder blades down and lift the chest naturally to create a positive outlook.

◆ If an exercise calls for a flat back, your spine should be straight and parallel to the floor.

◆ Lotus position: the classic posture for meditation and pranayama. Sitting with your spine erect, bend your knees and cross your ankles in front of you.

For the half lotus, pull one foot up high onto the opposite thigh and place the second foot under the thigh of your first leg.

For the full lotus, place the second leg over the first, with the foot high on the opposite thigh and your knees touching the floor.

The half lotus can also be assumed in a standing position and the full lotus can be performed sitting, or in the head and shoulder stands.

Safety guidelines

Here are some important guidelines which must always be followed in order to make sure that you are able to gain all the benefits that yoga has to offer and do not inadvertently injure yourself by exercising incorrectly.

◆ The yoga courses in this book have been designed for people who are in a normal state of health. As is the case with any fitness program, if you feel unfit or unwell or you are recovering from an illness or injury, are pregnant, have high blood pressure or suffer from any medical disorder you must consult your doctor before embarking upon any of the exercises.

Always follow the course exactly and do the exercises in the right order, and always begin your practice with the warm-up to help loosen the muscles. Exercising stiff muscles leads to injury.

◆ Never rush the movements and follow the directions exactly. Do not jerk your body and stop immediately if you experience any sharp pain or strain to any muscle.

Never push yourself and always do the pose only to your own capability. Remember that yoga is strictly non-competitive and, if you are following these courses with a friend, don't succumb to the temptation to go at the same rate of progress as him or her if it doesn't suit you. It is for you to find your own pace.

◆ Pay particular attention to your breathing in order to help relax and focus your mind. Pay special attention to your posture, too, and make sure that you always stand, sit or kneel upright (see pages 16–17).

When you are carrying out a standing exercise you will often be required to balance upon one leg. Keep the leg on which you are standing straight by lifting the muscle above the kneecap. Do not hyper-extend the knee because this can cause injury.

◆ Do not exercise on a full stomach. You must wait four hours after a heavy meal or one hour after a light snack.

◆ Choose a warm, quiet, well-ventilated place in which to exercise. Wear clothing that you can comfortably stretch in. All yoga exercises are done in bare feet so that you can grip the floor with your toes. You might need a mat for the floor work, but otherwise just make sure you exercise on an even, non-slip surface.

◆ After exercising, the body always needs a cooling down period to return it to normal. Always finish with the relaxation pose, even if just for a short time. However, the longer the relaxation period you can manage the better as deep breathing restores the equilibrium and calms the nervous system.

◆ Whenever you practice yoga, remember these basic principles: soul/mind control of movements; awareness of postures and movements; slow and deliberate movements; relaxation during movements; positive non-competitive attitude; go only as far as is comfortable.

Breathing

Learning the art of correct breathing is vital to your health and well-being. In yoga we breathe from the diaphragm. If you watch a baby breathe you can see the diaphragm rise and fall, but adults tend to breathe from the chest. When you breathe correctly you increase lung capacity and send more oxygen into the bloodstream, revitalizing and purifying the internal organs. Correct breathing acts as a natural tranquillizer to the nervous system; the deeper you breathe the calmer your mind becomes. Keep the breath even and always breathe through the nose, never the mouth unless specifically instructed.

1

Stand in perfect posture (see page 14). Inhale deeply and push your stomach out from the diaphragm. Do not move your chest, and keep your shoulders down.

2

Exhale deeply. Keep your breathing steady and even. Repeat Steps 1 and 2 for at least 10 full breaths. Always follow this breathing pattern before you start your yoga practice, to steady your mind.

Posture

One of the basics of yoga is to sit and stand in perfect posture, and many poses are designed to strengthen the muscles in the lower back so that you are able to lift your spine in perfect alignment. Whether you are sitting, standing or kneeling, think of a string pulling you up from the crown of your head. Always 'open the chest' by pushing your shoulder blades down, lifting the chest naturally. The basic standing pose is called Tadasana, which means 'the mountain'. It is a dynamic pose and you should be aware of every muscle in the body. Stand with your feet together and your weight evenly distributed between your toes and heels. Pull your stomach in, tuck your buttocks under and lift the muscle above the kneecaps. Keep your arms at your sides, elbows straight and fingertips together. To test yourself, balance on your toes; you should not fall backward or forward.

1

Stand tall with your feet firmly planted on the ground and your weight evenly distributed between your toes and heels. Keep your shoulders down and your stomach and tail bone pulled in.

2

Sitting cross-legged, lift your spine as far as you can. This will center your balance and create a positive mental attitude.

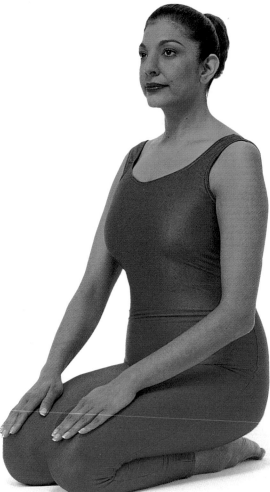

3

Sit on your heels and place your hands on your knees. Now raise your spine, straightening your elbows.

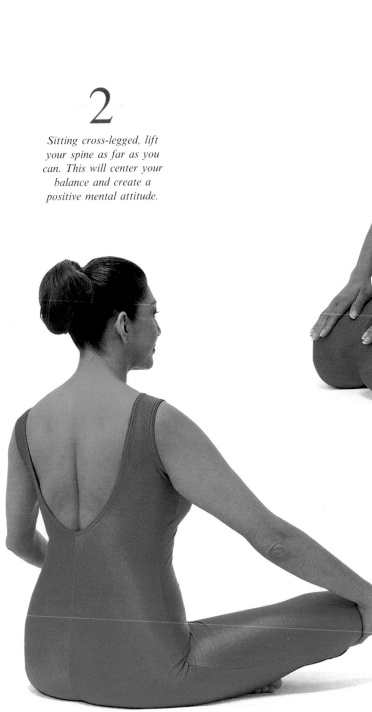

Warm-Up

It is always essential to warm up the body slowly and gently before beginning the yoga course of your choice. This series of movements combined with breathing in the correct manner will help to loosen the spine and gently prepare your body for the other exercises that follow. Before you begin, focus attention on yourself and breathe deeply from your diaphragm for ten seconds. 'Center' – that is, focus on balancing your physical and mental state – by assuming a good posture. You need to stand evenly with your weight balanced between your toes and heels. As you do the exercises you will feel the energy flow freely from one movement to the next.

1

Clasp your fingers together and raise your hands up to your chin. At the same time raise your elbows until they are even with your shoulders. Keep your head and chin raised.

2

Inhale and breathe deeply, bringing your elbows down toward each other. Make sure you don't drop your chin. Exhale and return to Step 1.

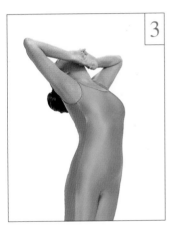

3

Drop your head back, raise your elbows and clasp your hands under your chin.

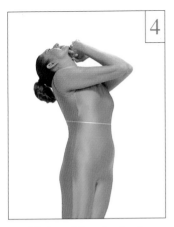

4

Inhale and breathe deeply, bringing the elbows together. Exhale and return to Step 3.

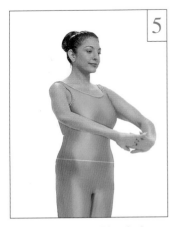

5

Bring your clasped hands down, inhale and then raise your arms above your head and exhale.

7

Put your arms down by your sides, then inhale and stretch your left arm over to the right, keeping the hips square. Exhale and stretch downward, extending the right hand toward the floor. Continue inhaling and exhaling and stretch in both directions for 5 seconds. Then repeat on the other side.

6

Keep your chin up and shoulders down as you stretch your spine fully by reaching your arms as high as possible. Slowly inhale and exhale.

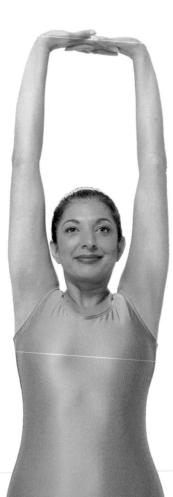

▶

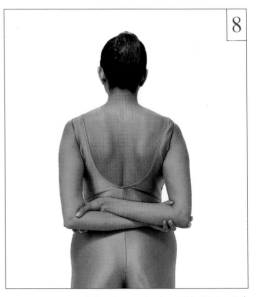

8

Put your arms behind your back and hold firmly onto your elbows with your opposite hand. Slowly inhale and exhale.

10

Exhale and lean forward so that your back is flat. Keep your spine straight and your chin forward.

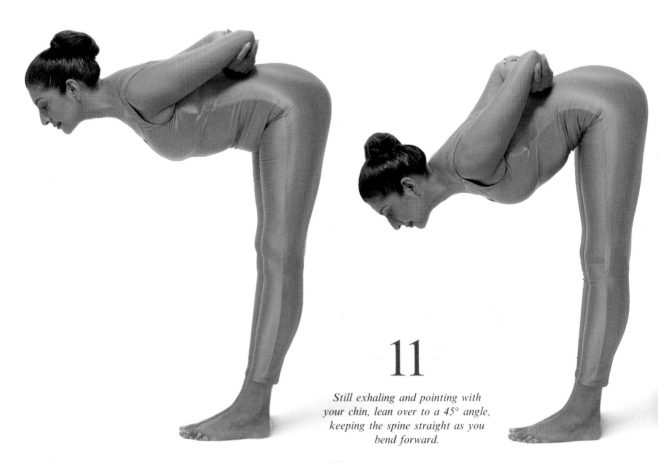

11

Still exhaling and pointing with your chin, lean over to a 45° angle, keeping the spine straight as you bend forward.

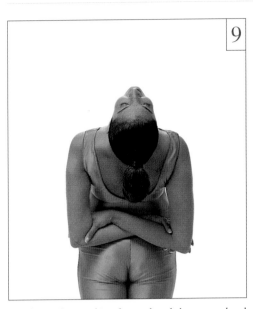

9

Inhale, push your hips forward and drop your head back, transferring your weight toward your heels. Keep your toes on the ground.

13

Inhale deeply and extend your arms out in front with your palms together and thumbs crossed. Keep your elbows straight and your arms close to your head. Inhale and exhale for 5 seconds.

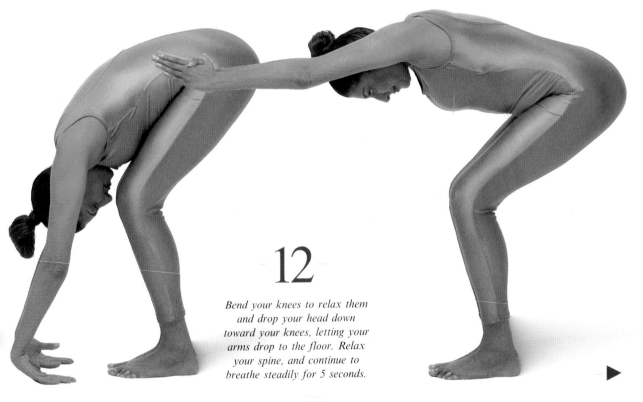

12

Bend your knees to relax them and drop your head down toward your knees, letting your arms drop to the floor. Relax your spine, and continue to breathe steadily for 5 seconds.

15

Inhale and as you exhale stretch all the way over to the right side. Keep your head evenly balanced between your arms and your feet together on the ground. Hold for 5 seconds, breathing normally. Inhale and return to Step 14. Repeat on the other side.

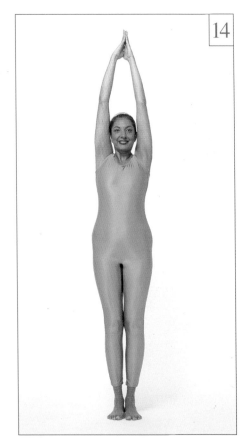

Return to a standing position, lift your arms high over your head and clasp your palms together.

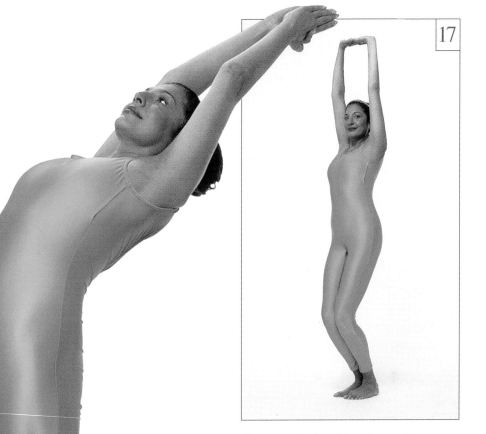

17

Return to the Step 14 position and keep your arms above your head. Now bend your knees, while breathing steadily.

16

Inhale and push your hips forward, taking the weight onto your heels. Keep your feet together, opening out your chest. Exhale. Lean backward as far as you can go. Breathe normally. Do not drop your head back, and keep your arms close to your head.

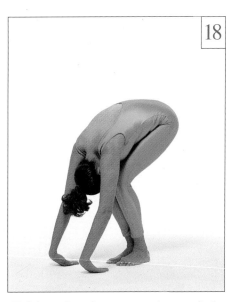

18

With knees bent, lean over to relax your body, dropping your arms down. Try to put your forehead on your knees. Uncurl and relax.

Relaxation

Learning the art of relaxation is essential to your well-being. These techniques not only help to rejuvenate the body but also release stress and tension in the muscle groups and calm the nerves. If you use the breathing exercise in the middle of the day it will refresh your mind and body. If you do it at night before you go to sleep, it can help cure insomnia. To release stress and tension in the muscle groups, begin by first focusing on your diaphragm and breathe deeply and slowly for 15 seconds. On every exhalation you'll feel the tension release from your body. Concentrate your mind on a pleasant image, such as a beautiful beach. Now concentrate on your feet and tense and release your toes. Flex your feet hard and as you relax them you'll feel the tension release in your ankles, knees, thighs, buttocks and stomach muscles. Repeat with your hands, tightening the arms and elbows while gripping your hands in a tight fist. Now raise your shoulder blades up and then relax them down again. Repeat twice. Next turn your head slowly to the right and slowly to the left, then let your head flop down. Finally, relax the face muscles, breathing deeply and keeping calm.

1

This is the dead man's pose. Lie flat on the floor with the palms of your hands facing upward and make sure your feet and legs are relaxed. Stay in this position for 15 minutes for the maximum benefit.

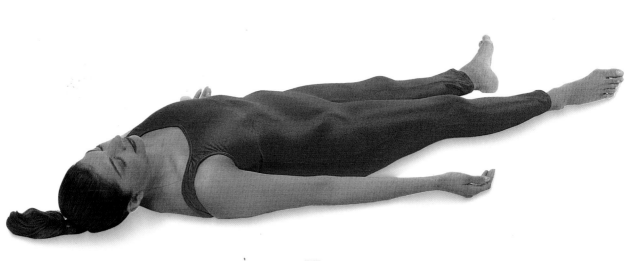

COURSE ONE

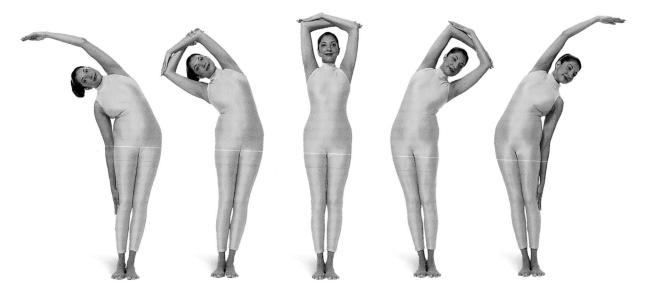

Course 1 is a foundation course for total beginners. It will teach you to balance your mental and physical energies and increase your flexibility and muscle tone, while improving your body shape and relaxing your nervous system.

Yoga is a science of movement: you should always begin with the Warm-up (page 16), and the exercises must be followed in their exact order. In Course 1 you are introduced slowly to the system with easy poses and stretches which will familiarize you with the yoga way of movement; you should pay special attention to details like hand and feet positions.

Remember that even when you do not feel as if you are moving, yoga is never static. Modern physical exercises like aerobics require a lot of energy, as every violent move burns it up; lactic acids are formed in the muscle fibers and this tires the muscles. The slow movements of yoga waste no energy; deep breathing allows more oxygen absorption and muscles suffer no fatigue.

Concentrate on what your body is doing. This is the first step toward disciplining the mind and body.

Head to Knee

This Head to Knee exercise lengthens the spine forward and is an excellent way to increase your body's flexibility and release unwanted body toxins. It helps soothe the nervous system, and will also relax the brain. You should never force your body forward, but as you increase the depth of your breathing you will be able to ease into the joy of deep stretching. It is very important to stretch forward from the waist. At the same time keep your back flat and don't round your shoulders. You might feel a pull in your hamstrings or some stiffness in the lower back. If this happens and you feel a bit dizzy, stretch your spine forward halfway, put your palms on a wall and keep your feet slightly apart.

1

Begin the exercise by standing up straight. Bend your knees slightly and place your hands on your waist.

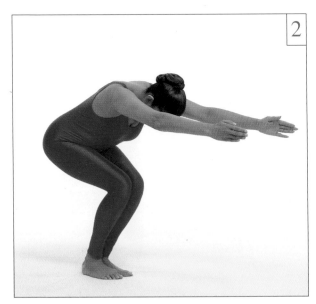

2

Inhale and throw your arms forward, putting your head down between your arms. Bend your knees deeper and keep your head in line with your back.

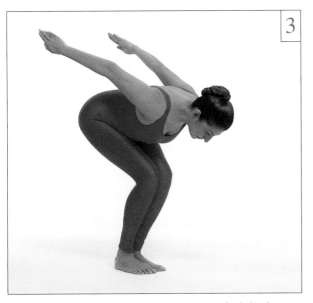

Exhale and then throw your arms out straight behind your back, in line with your shoulders, but still keep your body in the same bent position.

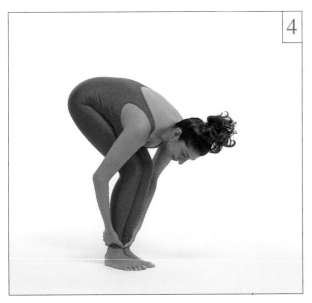

Take your hands down and hold your ankles from behind, moving your head down toward your knees. Breathe normally for 5 seconds.

5

Now straighten your knees as much as you can. Pull your stomach muscles in, and drop your head down to your knees. Hold this position for at least 5 to 10 seconds. You'll feel the energy flow in a circular motion from your toes up the spine to your head. Uncurl and relax.

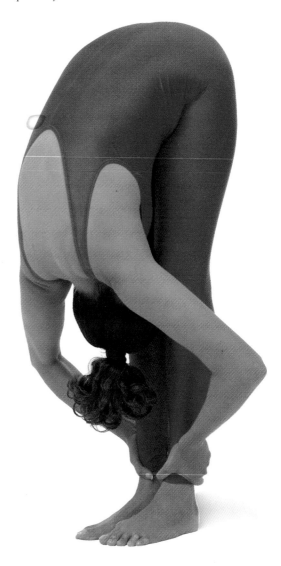

Dog Pose

This exercise is wonderful for stretching the whole body. Not only does it increase blood circulation, it also helps to tone and strengthen the legs and arms as well as curing fatigue and increasing your vitality. As with all the downward poses, it calms the nervous system and can be used as a relaxation pose if you're tired. Breathe deeply and evenly throughout the movements and relax your neck to release any tension in the shoulders.

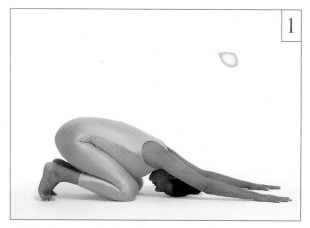

Sit back on your heels with your toes curled under. Stretch out your arms in front of you and straighten your elbows. Place your forehead on the floor.

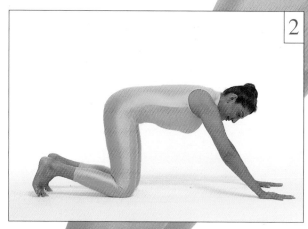

Inhale and kneel up, keeping your hands balanced out in front of you. Exhale and breathe normally. Stretch your fingers evenly on the floor, and keep your knees under the hips.

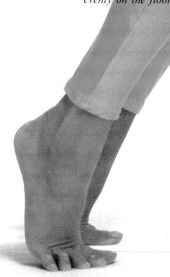

4

Now flatten your heels on the floor
and move your thighs outward. Lift
up your knees and stretch your spine
upward. Straighten your arms and
keep your shoulders down. Relax
your face and neck, and breathe
deeply for 30–60 seconds. As you
gain flexibility, hold for longer.
Relax and slowly stand upright.

3

Inhale, push the palms down and raise your
hips upward. Stretch high onto your toes,
pushing the shoulder blades down. Open out
the chest and release the neck and shoulders.
Bring your head in line with your spine and
push your hips back. Hold for 10 seconds,
while breathing normally.

The Tree

This standing pose focuses your mind and helps you learn how to concentrate and balance steadily on one leg. By balancing properly, you challenge your mind and you can unite your mental and physical energies. It also teaches you the importance of distributing your weight evenly between your heels and toes.

3

Now stretch your arms right up, while holding your balance for 5 seconds. Feel the energy move from your heels through your legs, into the spine and then through your arms and fingertips. Repeat on the other side.

1

Stand up straight. Place your right foot on your inner left thigh or close to the ankle or knee. Push out your hip but keep your hips square. Place your left hand on your left hip. Lift your standing leg as high as possible by stretching the muscle above the kneecap.

2

Look straight ahead and try to balance comfortably. When you are absolutely still, place your palms together and hold for 5 seconds. Grip the floor firmly with your toes so that the ankle does not move from side to side.

Side Stretch

Stretching to the side is an exercise that improves every muscle, joint, tendon and organ in the body. It also revitalizes the nerves, veins and body tissue by increasing the flow of oxygen to the blood. It helps cure sciatica, lumbago and other lower-back ailments. The body's strength and flexibility is heightened by the deep stretching, especially in the hip joints, waist and torso.

1

Stand up straight and place your feet about 1m (3ft) apart. Stretch out your arms with your palms facing down. Keep them in line with your shoulders. Breathe normally.

2

Turn in your left foot slightly and point your right foot 90° to the right. Inhale and stretch to the right. Keep the spine straight and do not tilt forward. Breathe normally and hold for 5 seconds.

3

Place your right hand on your right ankle and extend your left arm up in a straight line with your palm facing forward. Look up toward your arm, keeping your head up. Relax your face and shoulders, and hold for 10 seconds.

4

Take the left arm over and bend to the right to feel the additional stretch. Turn your head forward and keep your weight on your back heels to maintain an equal stretch on both sides of the torso. Hold for 5 seconds.

5

Return to Step 1. Bring your arms to your sides, placing your right arm on your right leg. Kneel on your left knee. Stretch the right leg out, pointing the toes. Balance evenly.

6

Inhale deeply and stretch out the right leg as far as possible without tilting forward. Stretch your left arm over to the right and feel the pull in your side. Keep your head balanced between your arms. Exhale and breathe normally.

7

Now sit on the floor, stretch out your right leg and fold your left leg in front, placing your foot on your inner right thigh. Clasp your right hand around your right foot and flex your thumb. Bend your right elbow and stretch forward toward the knee.

SIDE STRETCH

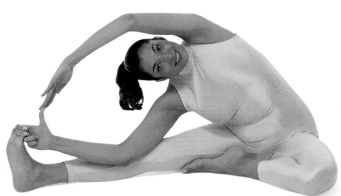

8

Inhale, take your left arm over your head and try to reach your right thumb with your fingers. Keep turning your upper torso to the side and keep your head evenly balanced. Increase the stretch and hold for 5 seconds.

9

Exhale and relax your head and arms down over your right knee. Keep your right foot flexed and, as you breathe normally again, relax your body further down toward the floor.

10

Lift your head up and stretch your legs out as wide as possible. Inhale and as you exhale stretch forward with your arms to reach your heels, or just reach for your thighs, knees or ankles. Stretch with your spine straight. Breathe deeply and hold for 10 seconds.

11

Now relax your head down toward the floor. Stretch your arms out, while keeping the toes flexed. Breathe normally and turn your knees upward, but push down. Hold for 15 seconds. Repeat on the other side.

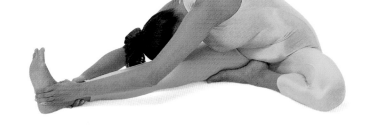

The Warrior

The Warrior pose is dynamic in its approach, and its aim is to develop a positive mental attitude and to give you physical control over your body. The Warrior is the basis for all standing postures, so the exact positioning of your spine, arms, legs and feet is very important. Hold your spine very straight as you open out your chest.

1

Stand up straight, feet together, and bend your knees slightly in preparation to jump. Bring your arms up to shoulder level and place your fingertips together.

2

Jump to open your legs wide – they should be about 1.2m (4ft) apart. Make sure your toes are pointing forward and stretch both your arms out sideways.

3

Turn your right knee and foot to the right. Lean your body backward and push your hips and stomach forward. Now bend your right knee, keeping your spine straight. Bend further until there is a 90° angle between your thigh and the floor. Repeat on the other side.

Side Twist

The standing twist helps to tone the leg muscles and waist, as well as relieving back pain and other ailments such as sciatica and lumbago. The twisting motion invigorates the abdominal organs and releases any toxins from the system. Remember to keep both legs straight as you twist from the hip upward.

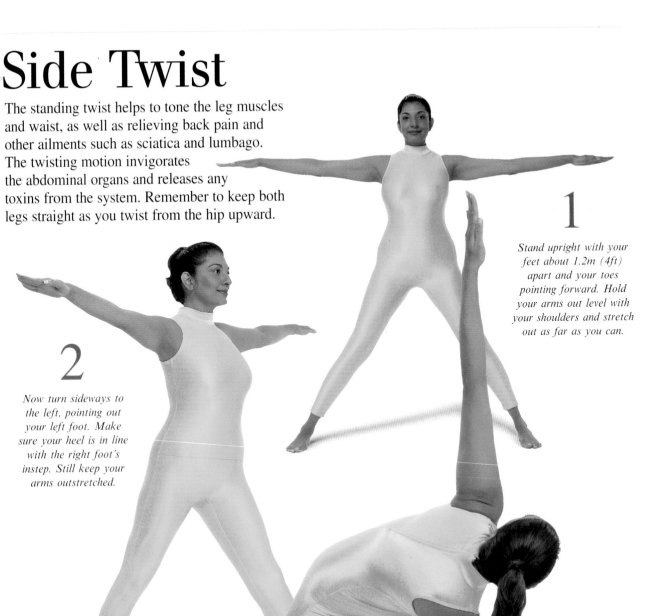

1

Stand upright with your feet about 1.2m (4ft) apart and your toes pointing forward. Hold your arms out level with your shoulders and stretch out as far as you can.

2

Now turn sideways to the left, pointing out your left foot. Make sure your heel is in line with the right foot's instep. Still keep your arms outstretched.

3

Now hold your left ankle with your right hand and look over your left shoulder. Keep your arms in a straight line. Hold for 10 seconds and then repeat on the other side. Breathe normally throughout.

Sitting Twist

If you practice these twisting movements regularly, any pain that you are suffering in your lower back will rapidly diminish. The muscles of your neck will also be strengthened, especially when you look over the shoulder (not shown) and any tension is released from your spinal system. Your liver and spleen are activated by the movements and the size of your abdomen is reduced in the twisting position.

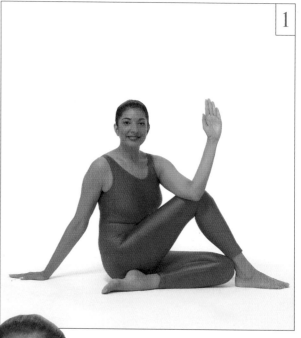

1

Sit on the floor and bend your left leg flat in front of you with your knee in direct line with your left hip. Take your right leg over your left leg, placing your right heel in front of your left knee. Take your left elbow over your right knee and twist to look over your right shoulder. Place your right hand lightly on the floor for support. Sit upright to twist your spine further.

2

Repeat the exercise on the other side. Make sure the palm of your raised arm is facing up with the fingertips together.

Toe Pull

This Toe Pull exercise stretches the body forward from the hips, helps to strengthen the leg muscles and increases the flexibility of the hamstrings and the spine. The movement stimulates the kidneys, liver and pancreas as you pull in the abdominal muscles. It also helps to flatten the stomach.

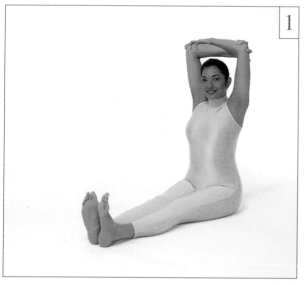

Sit upright with your legs out in front of you. Flex both feet and raise your arms over your head. Hold onto your elbows, keeping your shoulders down. Breathe normally.

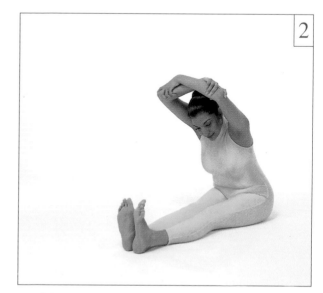

Bend forward from the hips, keeping the back flat. Try not to curve your spine. Hold up your chin, keeping your head balanced between your arms. Hold for 5 seconds.

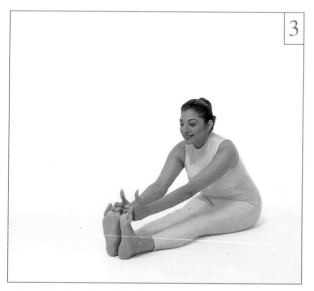

Reach further forward and try to grasp two fingers around your big toes. Flex the thumbs and keep the elbows straight. Inhale and exhale, and hold for 5 seconds.

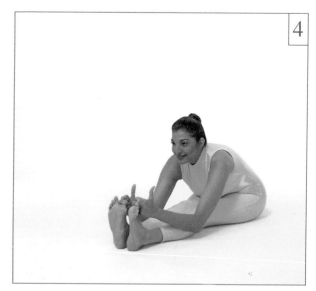

Bend your elbows and stretch forward, pointing your chin. Keep your back flat and your head out in front. Breathe deeply and hold for 10 seconds.

Leg Pull

1

Lie balanced on your side, leaning on your left elbow. Make sure your elbow is directly under your shoulder blade. Point your toes.

This exercise improves the flexibility of the leg muscles and also helps to tighten the abdominal muscles. The lower back is strengthened, and the movements help to give you good balance. Sit upright as much as possible to avoid rolling over to one side.

2

Inhale and bend your right knee in at a 90° angle to your left leg. Take hold of your big toe with your right hand and flex your thumb. Exhale.

3

Inhale and straighten your right leg to make a 90° angle with your left leg, flexing the toes. Breathe normally and hold for 5 seconds. Relax the leg down and repeat on the other side.

Flat Twist

The Flat Twist relieves any tension that gets trapped in the neck and shoulders. It also alleviates lower back pain and is a really good stretching exercise for your spine. Remember to keep both shoulders flat on the ground and always look in the opposite direction to your feet to increase the body stretch.

1

Lie flat on the ground and take your arms out to the side, placing your palms facing down. Put your left heel on top of the toes of the right foot. Breathe normally.

2

Inhale and as you exhale twist both feet to the right and look over your left shoulder. Hold the position for 5 seconds.

3

Bend your knees into your chest to increase the stretch, keeping legs and feet together. Inhale as your legs come up and then exhale and twist to the left. Relax onto your back and repeat on the other side.

Leg Lifts

These exercises will tone your stomach and leg muscles and improve the flexibility of your hamstrings and spine. It might be quite difficult in the beginning to achieve Step 3, but with continued practice you will be able to release all the stiffness in your joints.

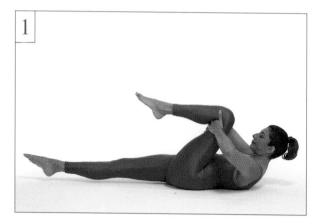

Lie on the floor. Clasp your hands behind your left knee and bring it into your chest. Lift your head up from the floor toward the knee. Point your toes and lift your right leg just off the floor. Breathe normally and hold for 5 seconds.

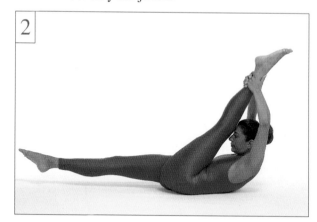

Put your hands around your ankle, if you can, and stretch further, trying to place your forehead on your knee. Trying to keep both legs straight and breathing normally, hold for 10 seconds. Repeat Steps 1 and 2 on the other side.

3

Clasp your fingers around your big toe and pull your right leg even further toward your head, keeping your right foot flexed. Take your left arm out, with your palm facing down, and hold just above your left leg. Breathe deeply, hold for 10 seconds and repeat on the other side.

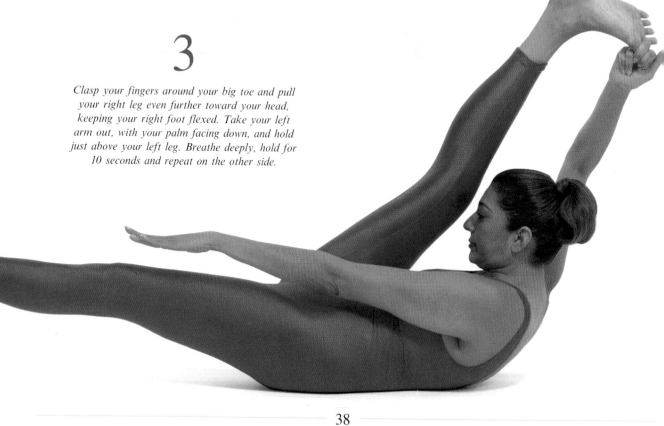

The Fish

When you do the Fish exercise you'll tone the stomach and leg muscles as well as releasing tension in the neck and shoulders. It also improves circulation to the face and slows the ageing process. These movements strengthen the lower back and open out the chest, increasing your lung capacity, which improves conditions such as bronchitis and asthma.

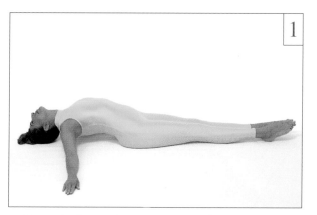

1

Lie on the floor with your arms out and point your toes. Inhale and raise your chest, resting your weight on the crown of your head. Feel the stretch in your neck and face. Exhale and breathe normally, holding for 3 seconds.

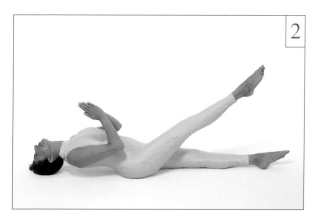

2

Still balancing on your head, inhale and raise your right leg, keeping your hip on the floor. Place your palms together above your chest, holding for 3 seconds. As you exhale, lower your leg slowly. Relax to the floor, if necessary, before Step 3.

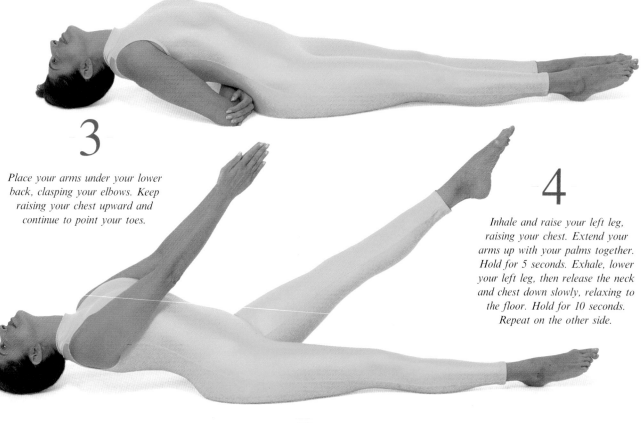

3

Place your arms under your lower back, clasping your elbows. Keep raising your chest upward and continue to point your toes.

4

Inhale and raise your left leg, raising your chest. Extend your arms up with your palms together. Hold for 5 seconds. Exhale, lower your left leg, then release the neck and chest down slowly, relaxing to the floor. Hold for 10 seconds. Repeat on the other side.

Back Bend

All back bends strengthen the spine and open
out the chest cavity to improve deep breathing.
The movement increases blood circulation and
raises energy levels. Even though back bends
are strenuous to do, it is very important to keep
your face relaxed and free of tension
throughout. You will feel exhilarated in Step 4
as your whole body, especially your arms and
legs, is strengthened. The deep breathing
technique will also give you a feeling of
complete calm.

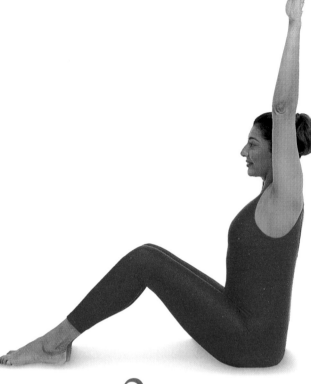

2

*Inhale and sit up tall, stretching your
arms upward in line with the side of
your head. Stretch out your legs
slightly, but keep your feet together.
Breathe normally.*

1

*Lie flat on the floor and bring your
knees up. Place your feet as close to
your body as possible. Stretch both
your arms out behind your head and
breathe normally.*

3

Keeping your feet flat on the floor, balance your arms behind you. Place your palms in opposite directions to your feet to support your body weight. Inhale and lift your buttocks, keeping an even line between your knees, hips and shoulders. Look up, exhale and breathe normally for 5 seconds.

4

Inhale, extend your legs and straighten your knees. Drop your head back and relax the neck and face. Keep pushing your hips upward. Breathing normally, hold for 5 seconds.

The Cobra

The Cobra strengthens and tones the lower back muscles. It alleviates back pain and prevents other common back ailments. The action of The Cobra tightens the buttock muscles and increases the intra-abdominal pressure which tones the uterus and ovaries. It also regulates the menstrual cycle and helps the thyroid and adrenal glands to work more effectively.

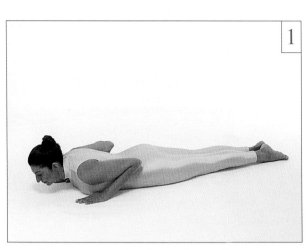

Lie flat on your stomach with your feet together. Point your toes, bend your arms close to your body, and place your palms flat under your shoulder blades. Point your chin downward.

2

Inhale and raise your head off the floor. Place your hands on the floor with your elbows inward. Keep your chin up and make sure your hip bones stay on the floor. Breathe normally and hold for 10 seconds. On the last exhalation, slowly lower yourself to the floor and return to Step 1. Repeat.

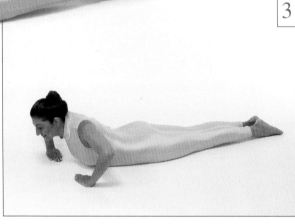

Return to Step 1, but this time place your hands under the breastbone and point your elbows outward.

4

Inhale, push down and lift your body off the floor. Look upward, keeping your shoulders down and your hips just off the floor. Breathing normally, hold for 10 seconds. On the last exhalation, slowly lower yourself and relax.

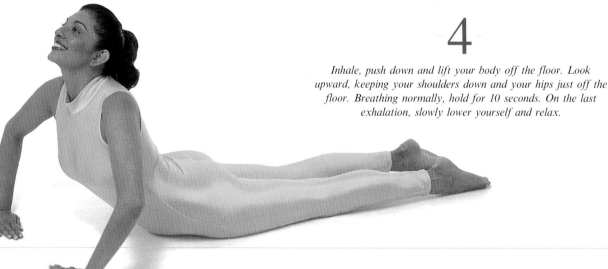

Back Lift

This exercise is rather strenuous to do and your body needs to be correctly aligned to achieve the right results. Not only does this type of lift tone the legs, buttocks, and stomach muscles, it also strengthens the lower back to enable you to sit and stand with perfect posture. Both your hip bones and shoulder blades should remain on the floor to stop you moving from side to side throughout the exercise. As a beginner you need not worry about the height of your leg lift, but as you gain strength and continue practicing, your hips will become more flexible and you will be able to lift your legs even higher.

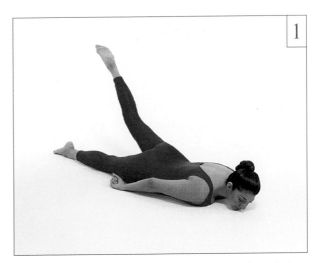

Lie on the floor face down. Keep your back straight and place your arms by your sides, holding your hands as fists. Inhale and raise your left leg, keeping your hips square. Breathe normally and hold for 6 seconds. On the last exhalation slowly lower the leg, then inhale and repeat on the other side.

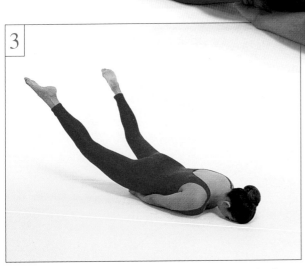

2

With your feet together, raise your hips slightly off the floor with your elbows resting under the hip bones. Keep your hands in fists, balanced under the thighs for support.

Inhale and raise your legs. Place your forehead on the floor. Keep lifting, breathing deeply, for as long as you can. On the last exhalation lower both legs. Repeat, then turn your head to one side and relax.

Cat Stretch

This is a wonderful body stretch to release tension trapped in the spine. It is excellent if you are very tired, as it invigorates the nervous system and helps calm the mind. If you are experiencing any back pain this is the best way to ease it. This is a relaxed pose, so you can hold it for as long as you wish. Inhale and exhale deeply to increase the calming effect.

1

Lie flat on the floor and bend your arms, keeping your hands under your shoulder blades. Point your toes and relax your elbows, but hold them close to your body.

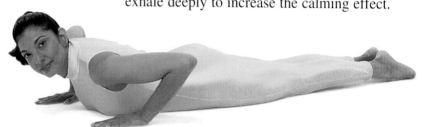

2

Inhale deeply and push down on your palms so that you can lift your hips upward into a kneeling position just like a cat.

3

Exhale and stretch your hips back so that you sit on your heels. Straighten your elbows, stretching your arms out in front of you. Place your forehead on the floor. Breathe normally and relax.

Soles of Feet

This Soles of Feet movement opens up the hips and increases flexibility in the hip joints, knees and thighs. Rotating the legs outward helps to increase the body's suppleness and also improves overall posture and mobility of the spine. It is an ideal exercise to do in preparation for giving birth, but take care not to bounce or jerk the spine.

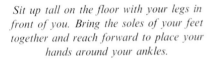

1

Sit up tall on the floor with your legs in front of you. Bring the soles of your feet together and reach forward to place your hands around your ankles.

2

Bring the heels closer into your body and sit upright. Relax your shoulders, then stretch up from the pelvis and open out the chest.

3

To increase the stretch of the hips, thighs and knees, place your elbows over the knees. Bend over, curving your spine and keeping your shoulders down. Inhale, and as you exhale push your knees to the floor. Breathe and relax into the stretch, slowly lowering your head to your feet.

Breathe and Relax

Stretching out the body is the best way to release any stress in your muscles. Combining stretching movements with deep breathing helps to calm and relax the nervous system. It also increases energy levels, flexibility and suppleness of the muscles, and gives a sense of physical and mental well-being. Never force your body through the exercise – use gentle movements, flowing into each position. You will soon appreciate the rejuvenating joy and challenge of deep stretching.

1

Sit on the floor with your legs wide apart. Flex your toes upward and try to push your knees down to the floor. Clasp your fingertips together in front of you.

2

Inhale, lean forward and stretch your arms out, keeping your hands up over your head. Turn your thighs outward to increase the stretch.

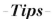

-Tips-

◆ *Don't force yourself into the stretches for this exercise, but as you become more supple, try pushing yourself a little further forward or upward.*

4

Exhale, drop your head back and look up to your clasped palms. Do not cave in at the chest or release your lower back. Inhale again and return to Step 3.

3

Continue to inhale and raise your arms up high over your head. Sit as tall as you can and open out your chest, keeping your shoulders down.

▶

5

Inhale and as you exhale stretch over to the right, keeping your spine straight. Breathe normally and hold for 5 seconds. Inhale and then return to Step 3.

6

Exhale and stretch over to the left. Try to balance your head evenly between your arms. Breathe normally and again hold for 5 seconds. Inhale and return to Step 3.

7

Exhale as you relax forward onto the floor. Keep your toes flexed and try to place your forehead right on the floor. Inhale and exhale deeply for 20 seconds and relax into the stretch.

Pranayama

'Prana' is the Sanskrit word for energy and 'pranayama' is the yoga breathing technique that unblocks this flow in the body and balances the masculine and feminine energies. Breathing correctly from the diaphragm acts as a natural tranquilizer and calms the nervous system. Always breathe through the nose, and as you exhale you will find that your lung capacity is increased and that more oxygen reaches the bloodstream. This rejuvenates the blood cells and increases vitality.

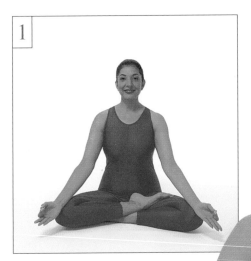

1

Sit cross-legged on the floor, or on a chair with your lower back supported, in which case keep your knees together and your feet flat on the floor. Place your thumb and first finger together and turn your palms upward. Focus on your diaphragm, and try to keep one thought in your mind. Breathe deeply, holding the position for at least 60 seconds.

2

To release tension in the neck and shoulders, inhale and raise your shoulders to your ears. Then exhale and lower them again. Repeat 3 times.

3

Return to Step 1. Drop your chin into your chest. Inhale and begin a full head circle to the right. Roll your head slowly, gently twisting your neck.

4

Take your head over to the right side, keeping your shoulders square to maximize the stretch. Keep your chin level.

5

Continue to inhale and drop your head all the way back behind you. As you exhale, roll your head to the left and complete the circle. Repeat on the other side.

COURSE TWO

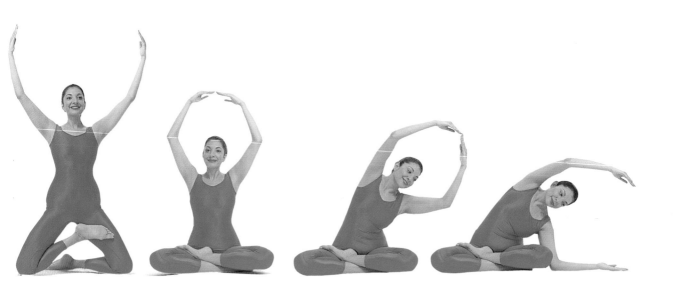

By now you have become familiar with the general style of yoga exercises and you have gained more flexibility, strength and stamina. You are now ready to twist your body in various ways, remembering, of course, to start with the Warm-Up (see page 16).

In Course 2 you will experience the energy flowing from one position to another. The muscles, joints and blood vessels will all be stretched, so that the blood is equally distributed to every part of the body and more energy flows into the relaxed muscles.

Try to hold the postures for longer with a calm and still mind. The only difference between a beginner and an intermediate student of yoga is the length of time a pose is held. This gives time for the mind to focus and the body to cleanse, purify and build the system.

Salute to the Sun

The Salute to the Sun is the classic warm-up exercise for all yoga practice. It increases the energy flow and improves circulation and muscle flexibility in the whole body. It also tones every muscle group, builds strength and stamina, and teaches you how to be graceful and well-poised. It is important to learn to move gracefully from one position to the next. Always breathe properly, because not only will your vitality level and energy increase, you will also feel rejuvenated and calm. While you practice the sequence, think of yourself as a dancer with total control over your body. As you become more supple, try to repeat the entire exercise up to 10 times on each side.

1

Stand up tall. Place your palms together in prayer position, keeping your shoulders down. Breathe normally.

2

Inhale and step to the right. Throw your arms back over your head and reach behind you. Push your hips forward, keeping your feet parallel and your toes pointed forward.

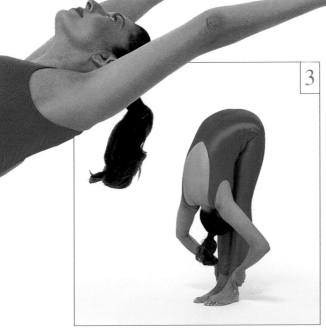

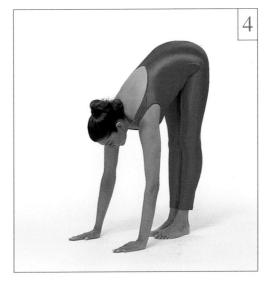

Exhale, step back with your feet together and bring your arms down. Stretch down to hold your ankles, pulling your forehead down to your knees.

Place your palms down on the floor in preparation for the next move. If you cannot keep your legs straight, bend your knees slightly.

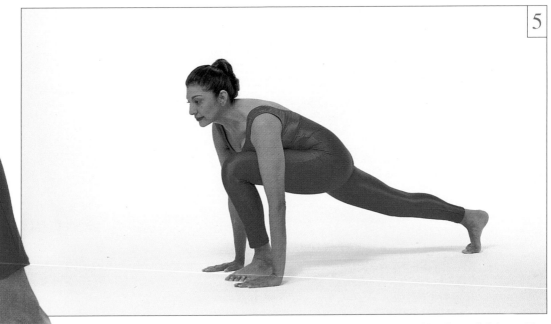

Inhale and take your right leg back behind you. Balance on your toes and bend your left knee. This is the position a sprinter adopts when preparing for a race.

▶

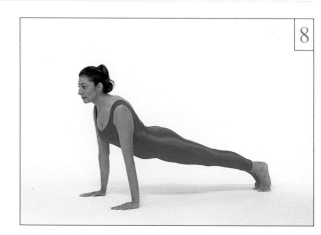

Leave your palms on the floor, inhale and stretch out both legs behind you. Keep your elbows straight and balance on your hands and feet. Keep your chin up and look forward.

6

Drop your right knee to the floor. Balance your weight at the top of your kneecap, but not on the kneecap itself, to prevent injury. Lift up your spine, raising your arms over your head with your palms together. Breathe normally and hold for a few seconds as you stretch.

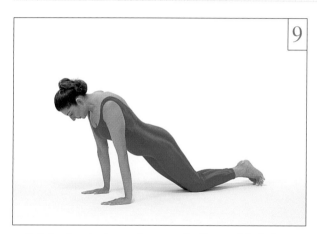

9

Exhale, drop both your knees to the floor and look down to your hands.

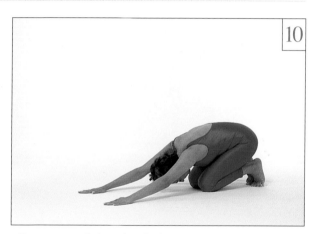

10

Continue to exhale and sit back on your heels, stretching out your arms in front of you to release your spine.

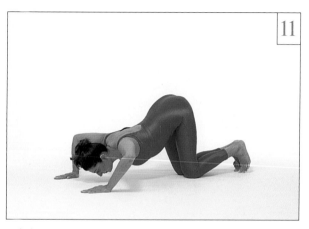

11

Inhale again and dive forward like a snake, keeping your chin near the floor to make your spine flexible. Bend your elbows.

7

Release down to the position for Step 5, and drop your head with your chin toward your knee.

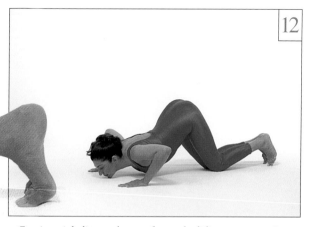

12

Continue inhaling and move forward, sliding out your chest and chin so that they are close to the floor.

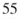

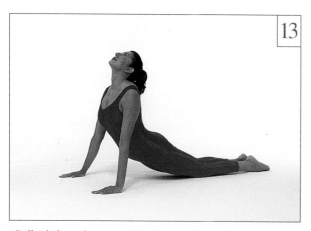

Still inhaling, drop your hips down and straighten your arms into the Cobra pose. Curve your spine, turning your head up.

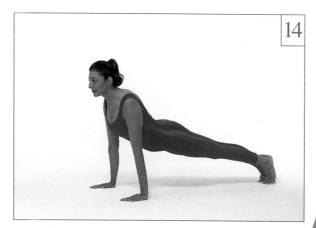

Exhale and return to Step 8, lifting your body up onto your toes again. Breathe normally.

15

Inhale and as you exhale, raise your hips, extending your spine. Keep your heels down on the floor and feel the stretch from your feet through your legs, spine, arms and into your fingers. This position is the Dog Pose. Breathe normally and hold for a few seconds.

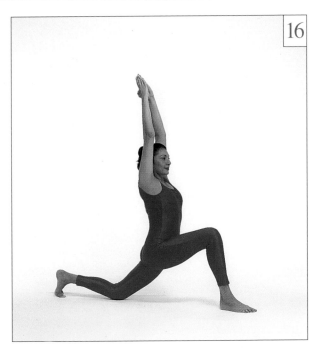

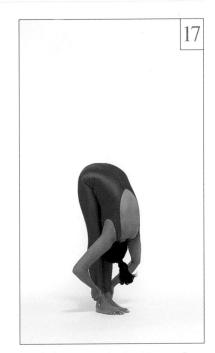

Return to the Step 6 pose, inhale, but this time bring the right foot forward and the left leg back. Hold for a few seconds and breathe normally.

Exhale, stepping back with your feet together, and bring your arms forward to return to the Step 3 position.

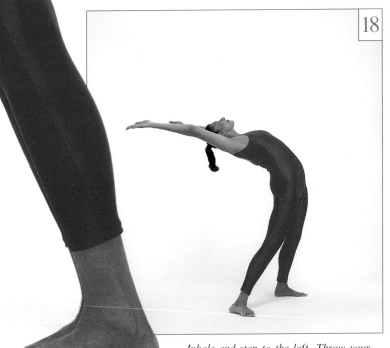

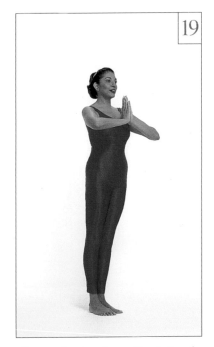

Inhale and step to the left. Throw your arms out behind you and bend backward as far as possible as in Step 2.

Put your feet together as Step 1. Breathe deeply, holding for 5 seconds. Repeat, using the opposite leg in Steps 5 and 16.

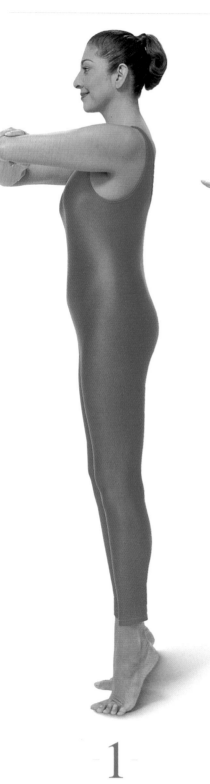

1

Stand up straight with your arms at your sides. Cross your arms in front of you and hold your elbows. Raise your heels and balance on your toes.

2

Straighten out your arms in front of you to help you maintain your balance. Bend your knees, keep your spine perfectly straight and try to hold still.

Knee Bends

These knee bend exercises build stamina and strength in the leg muscles as well as the abdominals. Balance is the key factor to doing them well, plus intense concentration. They help tone the spine as well as the calves, thighs and upper arms. The joints are also energized, which can prevent arthritis and rheumatism in the legs. These Knee Bends are grounding exercises which connect the earth's energy to the base of the spine. This energy then flows up the spine, increasing circulation and revitalizing your body.

3

Bend your knees down further so that you feel the extra stretch in your thighs, and keep lifting your heels upward.

4

Bend right down to a squatting position. Your knees, thighs and hips should be in a line at a right angle to the floor. Breathe deeply and hold as long as you can.

5

Stand up straight with your arms above your head. Cross your thumbs and put your palms together. Stretch your elbows, keeping your arms close to your head. Breathe normally.

6

Holding your upright posture, bend your knees but make sure that you keep your spine completely straight as you sink down toward the floor.

7

Inhale and take your hips back, making the movement from your tail bone. Adjust your weight to your heels and keep your back as straight as possible. Breathe normally and hold for 10 seconds.

The Eagle

The Eagle exercise focuses your mind so that you can concentrate on attention to detail. It grounds your energy and improves your balance. It can help to eliminate any cellulite and extra fat around the thighs, and also tones the leg, arm, and calf muscles. As you do the exercise, always keep your eyes fixed ahead on one spot to help you maintain your balance.

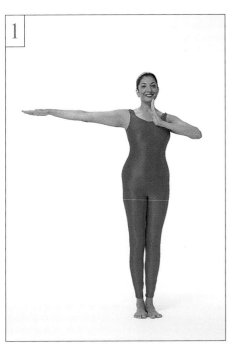

1

Stand up straight. Hold your left hand, facing upward, in front of your nose and stretch out your right arm. Focus on one spot straight ahead. Breathe normally.

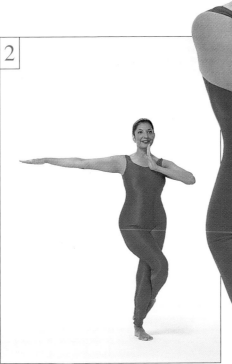

2

Bend both your knees and wrap the right leg around the left. Try to wrap the right foot around the left ankle. The deeper you bend the easier it is to wind your leg.

3

Bring your right arm under your left, crossing them at the elbows, but keeping your shoulders down. Twist your right hand toward your left palm in front of your nose and press palms together. Keep your shoulders even, but press down to open the chest. Breathe normally, holding as long as possible. Repeat on the other side.

The Letter T

Performing the movements for Letter T is very challenging and builds up your strength and stamina. It is a powerful and dynamic stretch and is the only asana that should not be held longer than 10 seconds. It increases your pulse rate and you will feel your breath coming more quickly. The stretching also firms your buttocks and upper arms.

3

As you exhale stretch out from your tail bone in both directions. Keep stretching your spine forward and keep pointing your toes behind you until you reach a perfect Letter T. Deepen your breathing and hold the position for up to 10 seconds. Repeat on the other side.

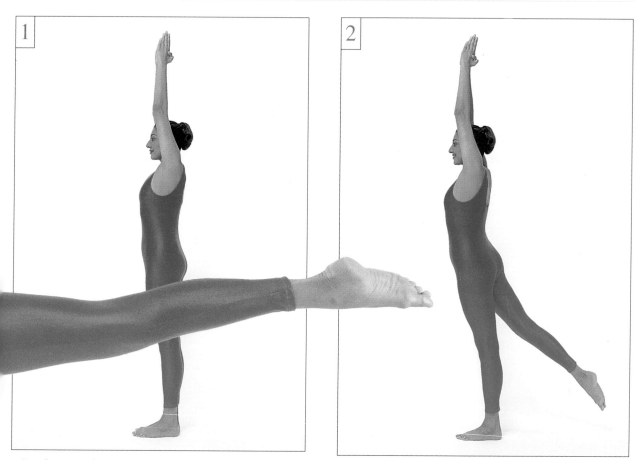

1	2

Stand up straight with your feet together. Raise your arms above your head. Place your palms together and straighten your elbows. Push your elbows back behind your ears, keeping your shoulder blades down. Breathe normally. | *Inhale deeply and point your right leg out behind you. Keep your right knee and your spine straight as you stretch out. Focus on one spot in front of you to keep your balance.*

-Tips-

◆ *It is important to breathe deeply from the diaphragm during the final position to increase your energy levels and vitality.*

◆ *Point your toes as much as possible. This will help to keep your knee and foot in a straight line.*

◆ *Keep pointing your toes and stretching your arms forward at the same time. Imagine you are a rubber band being stretched in opposite directions.*

Leg Extension

This position gives you more flexibility of the spine and builds strength in your lower back and legs. It opens the hips and makes you slimmer around the hips. It is also a difficult balancing exercise that focuses your concentration. The final position is quite hard to master, but don't get discouraged if you can't get your forehead right down to your knee.

1

Stand up straight with your feet together. Bend forward and grasp your ankles. Breathe normally.

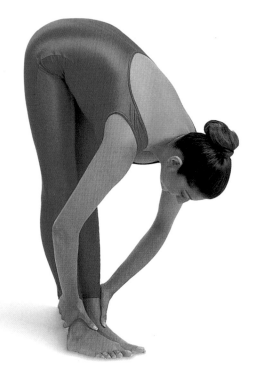

2

Place both hands on the floor in front of you and focus on one spot on the floor. Inhale and pull your stomach muscles up, while raising your left leg as high as possible. Keep the knee straight and point your toes. Breathe normally.

3

Still concentrating hard, take
your hands to your right ankle
and keep lifting the kneecap up.
Open your toes and grip the floor.
Breathe normally.

4

Keep stretching your leg out behind
you as you pull your head toward
your knee. Try to hold for as long
as possible, pointing your toes
upward, then slowly return to an
upright position. Repeat on the
other side.

The Tower

This series of movements increases the strength in your legs and also makes your spine more flexible. It expands the chest, helping you to breathe more deeply and improving your lung capacity. The exercise also helps to relieve any stiffness in the neck and shoulders and make them more supple. At the end of The Tower, when your head is resting on your knee, the abdominal organs are toned and cleansed – this is because your deep breathing has pumped fresh oxygen into the blood, increasing the circulation and revitalizing and purifying them.

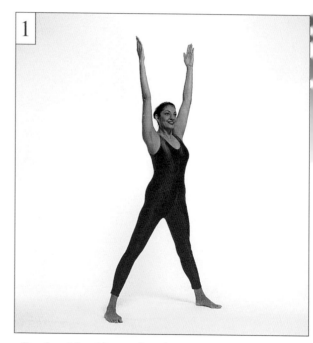

Stand upright with your feet about 1m (3ft) apart and your toes pointing forward. Take your arms up so that your palms face each other and straighten your elbows, keeping your shoulders down. Breathe normally.

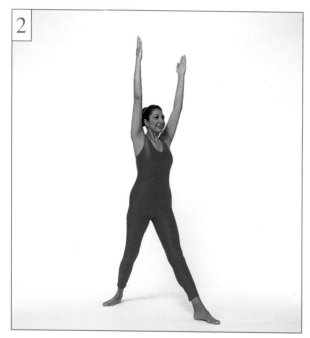

Turn your left foot to a 90° angle, while moving the right foot slightly inward. The heel of the left foot should be in line with your right instep. Keep your head evenly balanced between your arms.

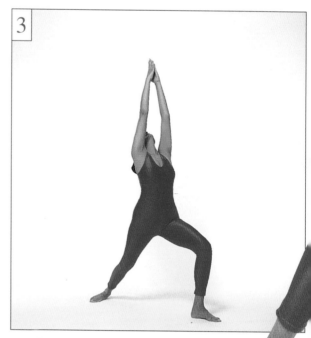

Bend your left leg so that your thigh is parallel to the floor. Throw your arms up and cross your thumbs with your palms together. Look upward and arch your spine. Breathe deeply and hold for 8 seconds.

4

Straighten your head between your arms
and move your body forward with your
weight on your left leg. Keep your leg,
spine and arms in a straight line. Breathe
deeply and hold for 8 seconds.

5

Relax down to the floor and
place your hands on the floor.
Drop your head to your knee.
Keep breathing normally.

6

With your head still at your knee and
with your palms on the floor, inhale
and straighten the knee as much as
possible. Breathe normally and hold
for 8 seconds. Return to Step 1 and
repeat on the other side.

Deep Lunge

The Deep Lunge exercises every muscle and tendon in the body. The intensity of the side stretch trims the thighs, hips and waistline, invigorates the internal organs and soothes the nerves. The position of the spine in relation to the hips helps to balance the endocrine system – the pituitary gland, thyroid, gonads and pancreas, all of which are glands that secrete hormones – as well as releasing toxins that build up in the system.

1

Adopt the Warrior pose (page 32), making sure your left leg makes a 90° angle and the back of your knee is in line with your heel. You can take the right leg further out to increase the lunge. Breathe normally.

2

Take your left hand down to your left ankle, turn your upper body and look over your right shoulder, twisting as much as possible. Place your right hand on the inner left thigh to increase the twist. Breathing deeply, hold for 8 seconds.

3

Place your left palm down
on the floor and extend
your right arm, elbow
straight, close to your ear.
Keep looking upward.
Breathing deeply, hold for
8 seconds.

4

Inhale and raise your body,
keeping your spine in the
same position. Clasp your
hands together over your head
and stretch upward. Breathing
deeply, hold for 8 seconds,
then return to Step 1.
Straighten the knee and repeat
on the other side.

Side Lunge

This series of movements increases flexibility of the spine, improves balance and tones and cleanses the abdominal organs. You may feel dizzy or nauseous during the exercise, but this is a good sign – it means you are releasing toxins in the system. Just stop if you feel in any way uncomfortable and breathe deeply to regain your equilibrium. Always stretch from the tail bone and keep your hips and torso square to the side.

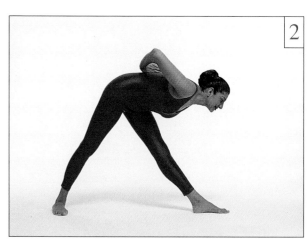

Exhale and, keeping your spine straight and your chin up, lower yourself to a 90° angle to the floor.

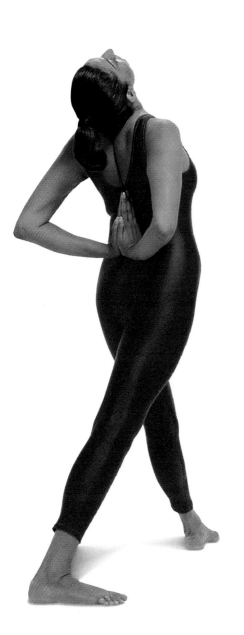

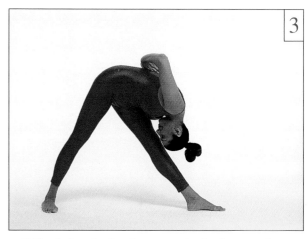

Still exhaling, bend and rest your forehead on your knee. Keep both legs straight – lift the muscles above the kneecaps to maintain balance. Breathing normally, hold for 6 seconds.

1

Follow feet positions in Steps 1 and 2 of Side Stretch (page 29). Place palms together behind your lower back or toward the mid-back. Push the elbows toward each other and open the chest. Look up and bend back as far as possible. Inhale deeply.

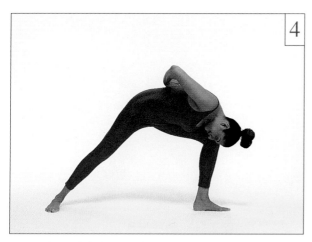

Bend your left knee and lunge forward. Drop your head down on the inner side of the knee. Breathe deeply and hold for 6 seconds.

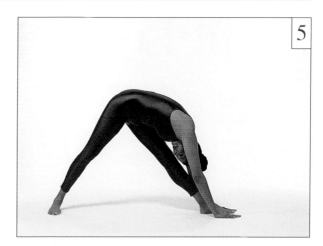

Straighten your knee, relax your arms down and place your hands on the floor, palms down. Breathe deeply and hold for as long as you can.

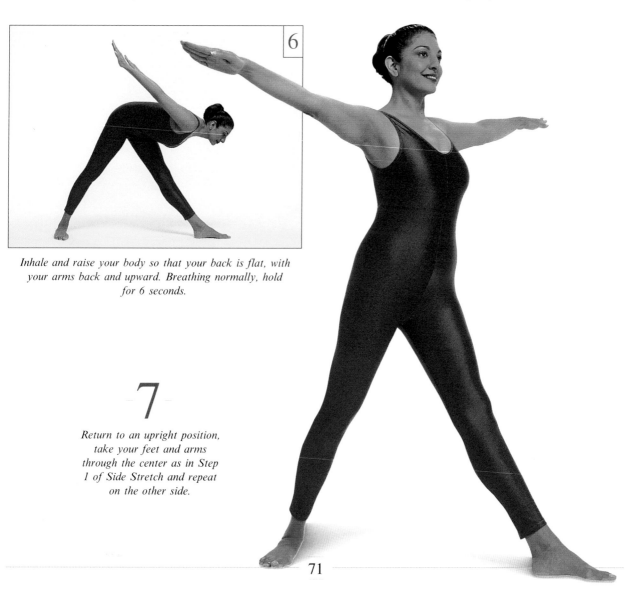

Inhale and raise your body so that your back is flat, with your arms back and upward. Breathing normally, hold for 6 seconds.

7

Return to an upright position, take your feet and arms through the center as in Step 1 of Side Stretch and repeat on the other side.

Front Lunge

This exercise is beneficial both mentally and physically. Stretching forward from the hips calms and soothes the central system, lifts fatigue, refreshes the mind and invigorates the blood circulation. The flexibility of the hamstrings, hips and spine is improved and the leg muscles are toned. Make sure that you always stretch forward from the tail bone and hold your stomach muscles up. Keep your spine straight throughout the exercise and breathe deeply from the diaphragm in order to increase the relaxing effect.

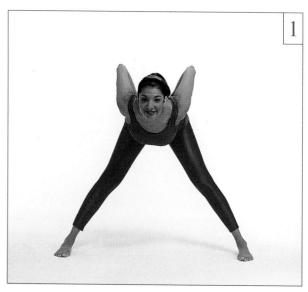

1

Stand tall with your feet 1.2m (4ft) apart. Place your hands on your hips. Inhale and as you exhale move your torso forward to flat-back position, keeping your chin up.

-Tips-

+ *Pay attention to your breathing, and take care not to hold your breath.*

+ *Push your weight onto your heels and grip the floor with your toes in order to steady your balance.*

+ *Keep your fingertips together in Step 4.*

+ *Whenever you straighten your legs, lift the leg muscles above the kneecap, to avoid injury.*

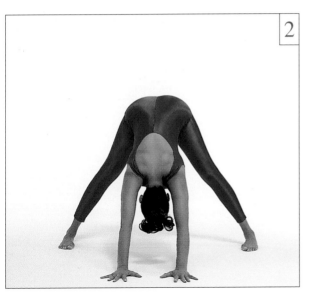

2

Still exhaling, relax forward, placing your hands on the floor. Push your weight to your heels, raise your hips back, grip the floor with your toes; open your fingers and stretch your spine.

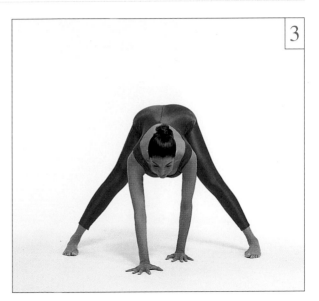

3

Walk your hands back and distribute your weight evenly between your heels and toes. Lift your chin and keep your back straight.

4

Inhale and raise your arms evenly on both sides. Keep your elbows straight and your fingertips together. Breathe deeply and hold for 6 seconds.

▶

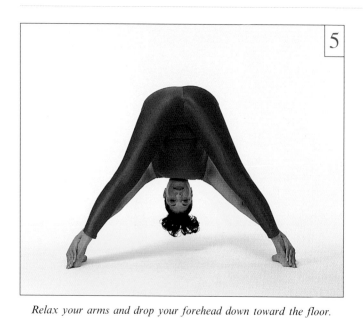

5

Relax your arms and drop your forehead down toward the floor. Breathe normally.

6

Inhale and clasp your hands around your ankles. Exhale and stretch your forehead down toward the floor. Breathe normally and hold for 6 seconds. Make sure your arms and legs are straight.

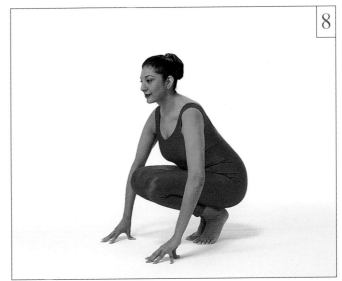

7

Bend your elbows and relax your knees. Push your palms down on the floor and prepare to jump into first position.

Inhale and jump. Breathe normally and balance on your toes. Steady yourself by placing your fingertips on the floor. Straighten the legs first, then the spine and stand in perfect posture.

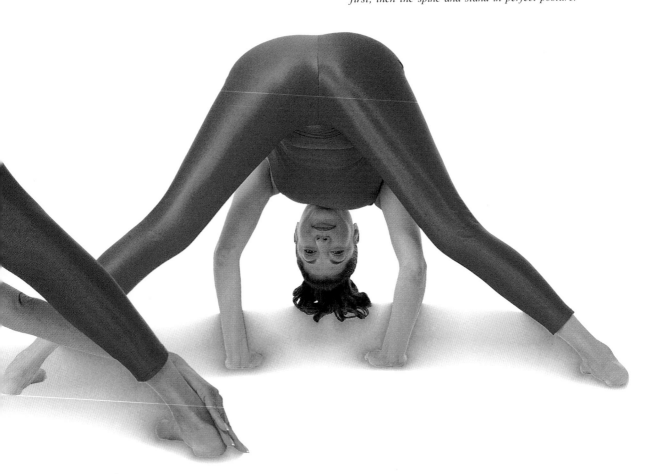

Toe Balance

The Toe Balance is an excellent way to improve concentration and confidence. All balances give you a sense of achievement, even if you are only able to hold the position for a few seconds. The most important thing to remember is that balance is a natural state of the mind and body which is lost as a result of the stresses and strains of daily living. These balancing exercises are designed to bring harmony to your total being and correct bad alignment caused by poor posture. You will know immediately when you are in correct alignment because you will feel a sense of joy and elation. Remember when you are trying to balance that it helps to focus on an object directly in front of you. Think of yourself as being absolutely still like a statue.

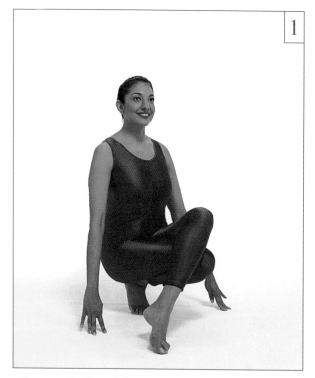

Squat on the floor, balancing on your toes with your knees together. Place your fingertips on the floor for support and cross your left leg across your right thigh. Keep your torso upright and breathe normally.

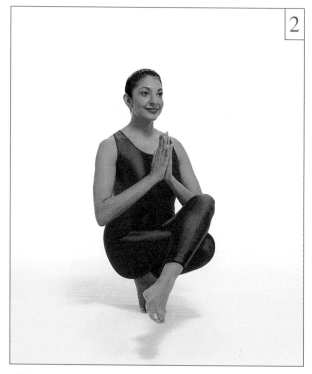

Focusing your gaze on one point, lift your left foot off the floor. When you feel totally balanced, bring your palms together and hold the position for as long as possible. Keep trying until you master the balance. Repeat on the other side.

Spinal Twist

The Spinal Twist opens the hip area, increases flexibility of the spine and releases toxins from the adrenal glands. It also tones the abdominal organs, kidneys, and spleen, aids digestion and cures digestive disorders. This pose stimulates the blood circulation to the spine and relieves backache. Because the abdominal wall is being contracted the abdominal muscles are stretched on both sides. When you are in the final position you will feel invigorated and energized.

1

Sit on the floor with both legs stretched straight out in front of you. Flex your right foot and take your left leg into a half-lotus. Sit upright and try to bring your left knee down to the floor. Breathe normally.

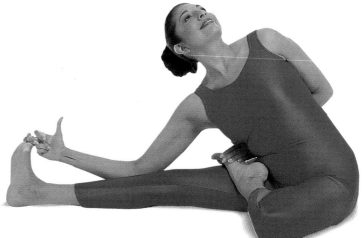

2

Reach sideways toward your right foot, bend your elbow and clasp two fingers around the foot, extending your thumb. Twist your spine and look over your left shoulder. Take your left arm around the lower back and take hold of the toes of your left foot. Keep twisting and turn your torso upward. Breathe deeply and hold for 10 seconds.

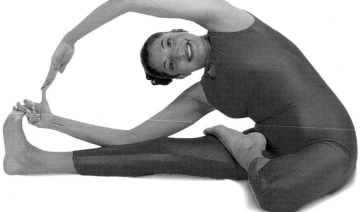

3

Release your left arm and take it sideways over your head to touch the right thumb. Keep your head even between your arms. Breathing normally, hold for 10 seconds. Repeat on the other side.

Sitting Balance

The Sitting Balance is an excellent test for checking your alignment – you will be unable to carry out this exercise if your spine is not in the correct position. Imagine your spine to be a group of children's building blocks; if you do not place each block evenly on to the next the whole building will come tumbling down. By the same token, if you do not lift your spine upright you will keep rolling back down to the floor. Concentrate on your stomach muscles because it is equally important to pull them in at the same time as you lift your spine.

2

Still sitting upright, bring your legs up to form an exact right-angle with the body.

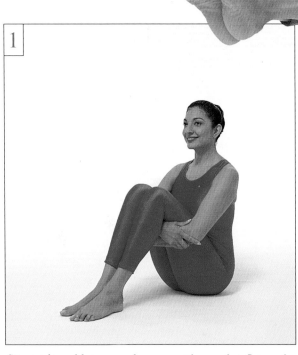

1

Sit upright and bring your knees up with your feet flat on the floor. Clasp your elbows under your knees. Keep your spine straight and breathe normally.

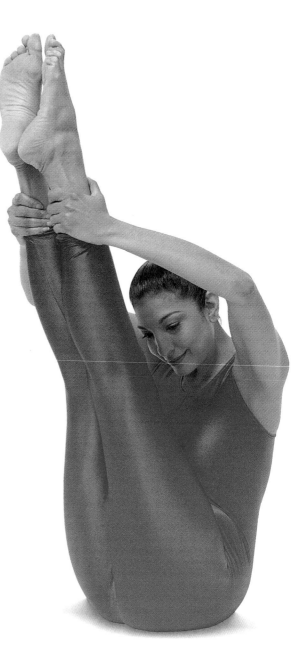

4

Shift your hands up your legs and take hold of your ankles. Pull your head toward your knees, keeping your spine straight and pulling your stomach muscles in. Breathe normally and hold for at least 5 seconds.

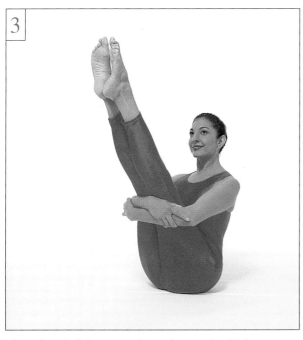

Straighten both legs up in front of you and hold the position absolutely still for at least 5 seconds, breathing normally.

The Plough

This is an all-body stretch that maximizes the flexibility of the spine and tones the leg and stomach muscles. The locking of the chin into the chest stimulates the thyroid gland, which regulates the metabolism and the hormonal levels in the body. Consequently, the Plough can help to cure an overactive or underactive thyroid and stabilize weight gain and irregular menstrual cycles. This inverted position unblocks energy, improves circulation and calms the nerves. Keep your breathing deep and even to achieve maximum benefits. Do not attempt inverted postures if you are pregnant or if you have a heavy menstrual period.

1

Lie flat on the floor with your arms to the sides, palms facing down. Inhale and, using your stomach muscles, bring your knees into your chest. Keep your shoulders down and relax the muscles in your face.

2

Exhale and throw your legs behind your head to the floor. Point your toes and straighten your knees. Keep stretching your legs and lock your chin into your chest. Breathe deeply.

3

To increase the stretch, tuck your toes under and clasp your hands together. Continue to breathe deeply.

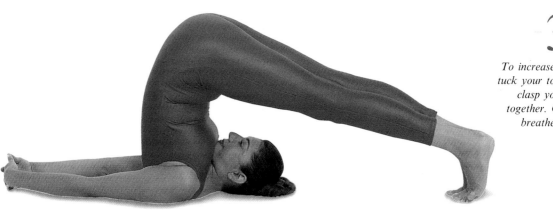

* If keeping the knees straight is difficult you can bend them slightly to avoid back strain.

* If you find difficulty breathing in the inverted position, descend back down to the floor, breathe deeply and relax. Resume the position when you feel ready.

5

To release the position, take both arms and legs behind you and place your toes into your palms. Close your eyes, breathe deeply and hold for 5 to 10 seconds.

4

Holding the same position, inhale and raise your right leg straight up. Point the toes and keep both knees straight. Breathing normally, hold the position for 5 seconds. On an exhalation lower the leg slowly and repeat on the opposite leg.

6

To relax the spine drop your knees to the floor, close to your ears. Take your arms down in front of you, palms facing down. Hold for 5 to 10 seconds.

7

To begin the descent back, lift your knees off the floor and place them just above your face. Point your toes and concentrate on your spine. Breathe normally.

8

Focus on your stomach muscles and lower back and slowly straighten your legs behind you, keeping the top of your spine on the floor. Breathe normally.

9

Exhale and, moving very slowly and with concentration, roll your spine down, working from the top vertebrae down to the tail bone without missing any sections. Return the legs to a right angle and hold for a few seconds, breathing normally. On an exhalation, using your stomach muscles, slowly lower your legs without raising your spine. Relax and breathe normally.

The Wheel

The Wheel, Bow and Camel are intense back bends that invigorate the spine, alleviate back pain and increase the lung capacity. We rarely stretch backward and these positions release fear and bestow a positive outlook on life. All three asanas release energy in the body's cells, glands and organs. The Wheel also builds muscle tone in the legs, hips, shoulders, arms, wrists and hands. Holding the position will build body strength and give stamina to the spine and limbs.

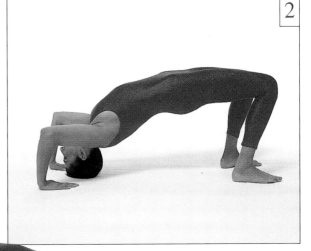

Lie flat, knees bent and in line with your hips, and feet flat and as close to the buttocks as possible. Inhale and raise your buttocks as high as possible. Try to hold on to your ankles. Breathe normally. Lower down and repeat.

Keeping your feet in the same position, lift your hips and buttocks and take your arms over your head with palms facing downward. Push up and rest on the crown of your head. Breathe normally and hold for 5–10 seconds.

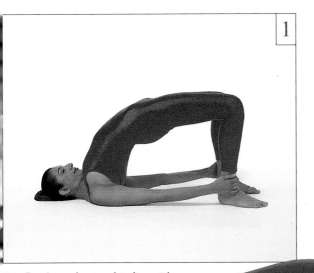

3

Lift as high as possible, balancing on your toes and hands. Straighten your elbows and, breathing normally, hold for as long as possible. Return to Step 2, lift your head toward your chest and lower your spine, one vertebra at a time, with your tail bone last.

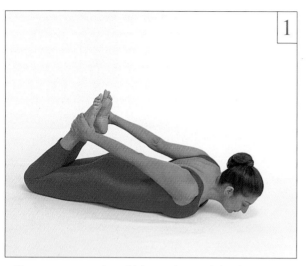

Lie on your stomach and lift your legs up behind you. Hold on to your ankles and point your toes. Place your chin and nose on the floor. Breathe normally.

The Bow

This exercise is called the Bow because of the beautiful bow shape that the spine creates. The back muscles and internal organs are massaged and the latter invigorated. Because of the position of the abdomen, this asana helps to cure digestive and bowel disorders such as gastroenteritis and constipation. It also stimulates the appetite, aids digestion and reduces fat along the stomach and middle of the back. As a result of the increased suppleness it gives to the spine every cell in the body is rejuvenated and revitalized, giving you renewed vitality and a more youthful appearance.

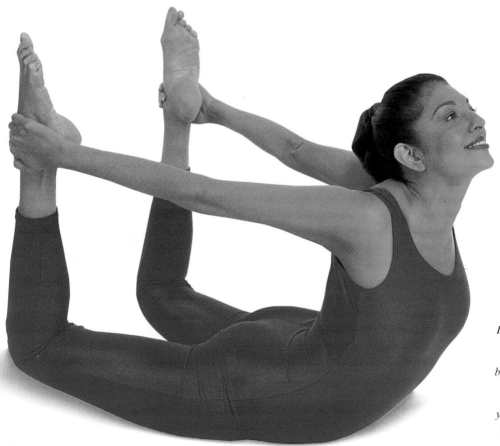

2

Inhale and lift your body up in one movement. Balance on your hip bones and keep stretching upward, trying to get your head in line with your feet. Breathe deeply and hold for as long as you can.

The Camel

The Camel tones the entire spine as well as every muscle group in the body, building strength in the lower back and alleviating back ailments, especially sciatica and slipped discs. It is also a wonderful stretch for the face and neck – the increased circulation helps to prevent the signs of ageing. Every time you do this exercise, feel your body giving way into the stretch and relax and open the throat and chest; do not allow any weight into the thighs or leg muscles. Always push upward from the hips to increase the intensity of the back stretch and breathe deeply throughout. If you experience a sharp pain in the lower back, stop immediately and relax in Step 3. A dull pain means you are using muscles around the spine that need toning.

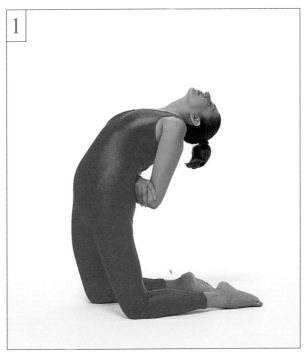

Kneel down, spine straight and hips directly above your knees. Hold on to your elbows behind your lower back. Inhale, push your hips forward and drop your head back. Breathe normally.

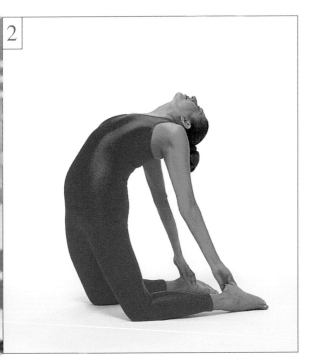

Continuing to push your hips forward, take your hands to your heels. Open your chest and throat and relax your face, neck and shoulders. Say 'Aah' in a clear tone to test that you are in the correct position. Breathe normally and hold for as long as possible.

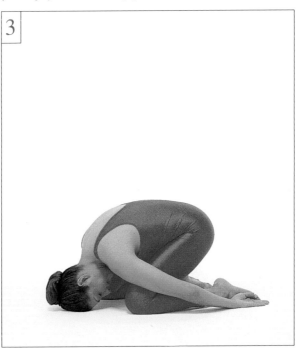

To release the spine, reverse the position by relaxing your head down to the floor with your palms facing up. Breathe normally and repeat the exercise.

The Rabbit

The Rabbit allows fresh oxygen into the blood supply, which stimulates and invigorates the brain cells. The upside-down position of the head has a beneficial effect on the pituitary gland and thyroid. It wards off senility, clarifies the mind, regulates the metabolism and strengthens the immune system. It also has a calming effect on the nervous system. A preliminary exercise to the Head Stand (page 124), the Rabbit improves the elasticity and mobility of the spine.

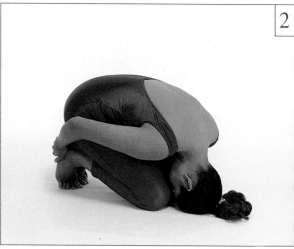

Inhale and as you exhale curl your spine and place your forehead on the floor as close as you can to your knees. Breathe normally.

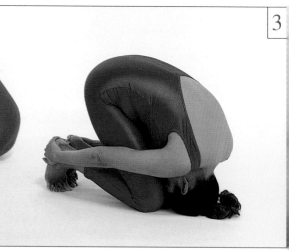

Roll on to the top of your head. Straighten your elbows and raise your hips. Breathe deeply and hold for 20 seconds. Return to Step 1 and repeat the exercise.

1

Kneel on the floor, toes tucked under your haunches. Clasp your hands to your heels and sit up tall. Breathe normally.

Eye Exercise

This exercise strengthens and tones the muscles in and around the eyes, increasing circulation and preventing wrinkles and fine lines from forming. It is also called the Clock because in doing it you visualize the numbers of a clock in clockwise and counter-clockwise fashion. Do not move your head but exaggerate the movement of your eyes. You may experience some strain but this is due to weak eye muscles; rub your hands together to make them warm and then cup your eyes to rest them. The shoulder stretch is optional, but it is a good companion to the eye stretch.

2

Keeping your chin level, look up at the number 12 of an imaginary clock. Focusing on each number, move your eyes clockwise, then repeat counter-clockwise. Repeat the exercise on the other side.

1

Kneel on the floor, tucking your toes under. Take your right arm over your right shoulder, placing your palm face down between your shoulder blades. Take your left arm around and clasp your hands together.

Pranayama

Pranayama are breath control exercises that allow the breath to flow smoothly through the seven chakra centers and unblock any negative energies. They also force the mind into intense concentration and traditionally are preliminary techniques to train the mind for meditation. Alternative nostril breathing balances the masculine and feminine energies which each of us has regardless of gender. It is vital for total mental and physical health to harmonize and balance these forces. The right nostril is the masculine side, so the breath will be deeper, louder and stronger; the left or feminine side will be soft, cool and quiet. As you inhale and exhale, concentrate on this and experience the difference between the breaths.

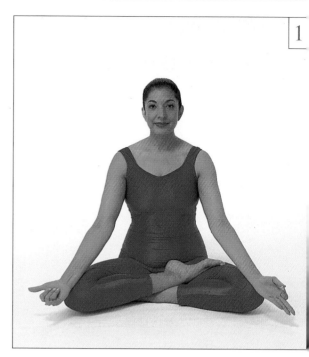

Sit cross-legged or in lotus or half lotus position, your spine upright. Touch your left thumb and first finger together and fold the three middle fingers of your right hand into your palm, extending your thumb and little finger.

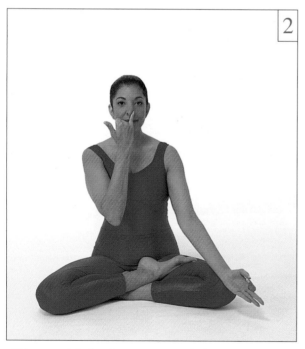

Take your right hand to your nose and block the left nostril with your little finger. Inhale and exhale deeply through the right nostril only. Continue for 10 breaths.

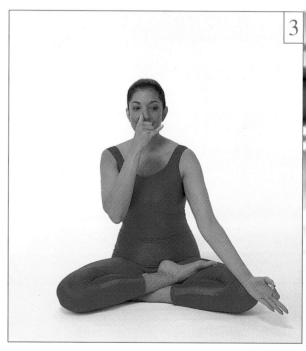

Block the right nostril with your thumb and breathe for 10 seconds. Repeat the exercise 3 times on each side. Finish by breathing through both nostrils as in Step 1.

COURSE THREE

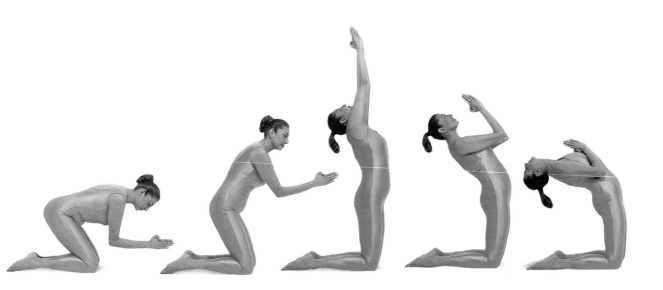

Course 3 is physically and mentally challenging and, as always, it is very important to warm up first. For you to enjoy these asanas you will need to have mastered the art of balance. At this level you will be totally centered and your approach to the asanas will be meditative. The exercises are dynamic and you will feel the energy flow from your toes through to your fingertips. Remember that the more energy you use, the more energy you will gain.

There is never a peak of perfection in any posture. Every time you begin an asana, challenge yourself to stretch further and hold the position for longer than the previous time.

Set goals for yourself and tell yourself that you definitely can and will improve.

Feel the stress leave your body as you twist and stretch. Think of your mind as the intelligent driver of a perfect automobile. You are the master of your soul and destiny and your yoga will take you to a new realm of calm, joy and contentment.

Vinyasa

Vinyasas are a series of different movements done in an active and dynamic style. Their function is to increase the stamina and strength of the body and to have an aerobic effect on the heart. Consequently, they are meant to be strenuous in nature and I have specifically designed this series to challenge your skill and to encourage you to develop grace through dynamic movement. Pay attention to the exact postures and do not rush. Breathe deeply and evenly through each of the positions.

1

Stand tall with your feet in second position directly under your hips and your knees bent. Inhale and throw your arms forward in parallel position.

2

Exhale, place your hands on the floor and jump, taking your feet out behind you. Stretch your spine and keep your legs and arms straight. Breathe normally.

3

Inhale, lift your heels and rise onto your toes. Change your foot position and balance on the front of your toes. Lower your hips toward the floor and raise your spine. Keep your shoulders down and look up. Breathe normally.

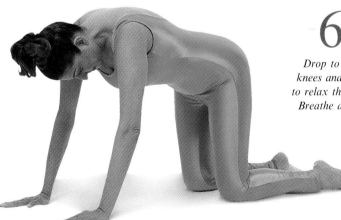

5

Exhale and place your left arm back down to the floor and swing your hips toward the floor. Tuck your toes under and point both hands forward and under the shoulder blades. Breathe normally.

4

Keeping your body in a straight line, turn your right hand to the front and your legs and feet together to the side. Raise your hips to maintain the straight line and raise your left arm, palm facing forward. Breathe deeply and hold for a few seconds.

6

Drop to your knees and begin to relax the spine. Breathe deeply.

7

Take your hips all the way back to your heels. Stretch your arms out in front of you. Breathe deeply and relax for a few moments.

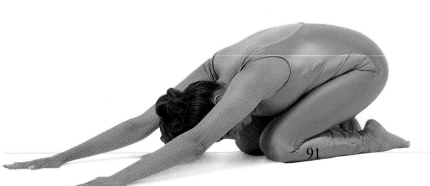

8

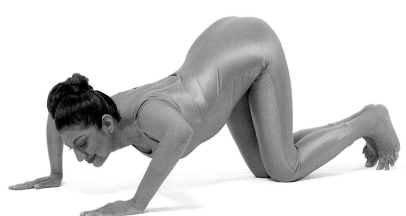

Keeping your hands in the same position, inhale and dive down, leading with your chin and moving your chest smoothly as close to the floor as possible.

9

Exhale, sweep the spine forward and come up into the Cobra pose. Breathe normally.

10

Inhale and return to the one-arm balance as in Step 4, but on the other side. Make sure your alignment is correct. Breathe normally and try to hold still for as long as you can.

11

Exhale and return to Step 5. Inhale and return to Step 2. Breathing normally, increase the stretch.

12

Inhale and raise your right leg in a straight line behind you. Point the toes, hold, and breathe deeply. Repeat on the other leg.

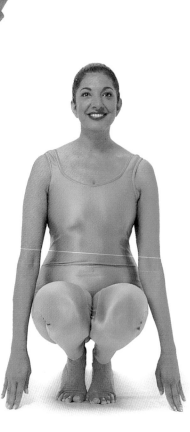

13

Walk your hands back to your feet. Bend your knees and balance on your toes. Straighten your spine and hold for a few seconds. Return to standing position and repeat the entire series.

Half Lotus

This exercise is a wonderful challenge because it combines balance with concentration. In all difficult standing postures it is essential to keep the weight-bearing leg absolutely still when progressing through the various movements. Make sure the leg is pulled up as high as possible by gripping the floor with your toes and lifting the muscle above the kneecap.

1

Stand up straight. Lift your right foot up and bring your heel as close as possible to the left hipbone. Breathe normally.

2

Push your right foot against your left leg and balance your weight on your left leg.

3

Bring the palms together to help focus your attention. Make sure your shoulders are down and your face is relaxed.

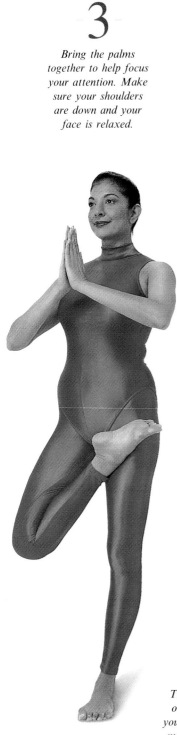

5

Release the foot and return to center position. Change legs and repeat on the other side.

4

Twist to the right and look over your right shoulder if you can. Having reached your maximum stretch, take your right hand around the back and reach for the right foot. Breathe normally and hold for a few moments.

Side Leg Stretch

This exercise looks simple but is in fact quite challenging. All the muscles in the legs are being toned and strengthened and suppleness is increased as you stretch to the side. The most important thing to remember is to keep the hips square. Open your chest without altering your posture and keep lifting as tall as you can. This position creates a positive attitude and the balance gives you steadiness and poise.

Tips

+ In all balancing exercises, keep your eyes focused on one spot as this helps to center your body and focus your mind.

+ If your ankle wavers from side to side during this exercise, grip the floor with your toes.

+ Do not collapse your spine forward when you clasp your toes in Step 2.

+ If you cannot stretch your leg completely in Step 3, bend your knee.

1

Stand up straight. Imagine a string is pulling you up from the top of the head to straighten your spine further. Put your left hand on your waist and use your right hand to lift your right leg up to the inner left thigh. Breathe normally.

3

Inhale, extend your right leg out from the knee and straighten your spine, taking care not to swivel your hips. Breathe normally and hold for as long as you can. Repeat on the other side.

2

Lean to the right, taking care not to twist your spine. Open your chest, clasp the two first fingers of your right hand around your big toe and extend the thumb. Breathe normally.

Head to Knee

This is the most difficult of the standing postures but it is well worth persevering with; not only does it build strength and stamina, it energizes the body, increases the flexibility of the spine and tones the lower region of the spine and the nerves connected to the legs. It also tones every muscle in the body, massages the internal organs and cures gastric problems. This is an excellent exercise for those who suffer from arthritis of the knees. It is important to hold the position for a length of time to allow the energy to flow in a circular motion throughout the system to improve circulation.

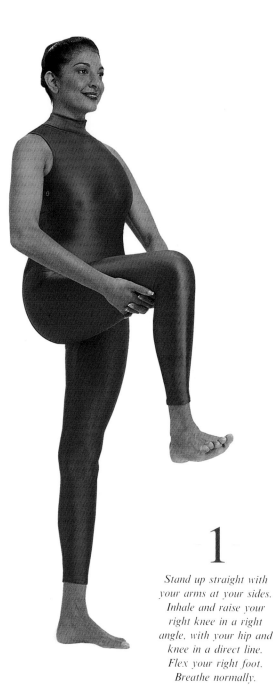

1

Stand up straight with your arms at your sides. Inhale and raise your right knee in a right angle, with your hip and knee in a direct line. Flex your right foot. Breathe normally.

2

Keeping your knee in a direct line with your hip, take hold of your right foot and pull it back. Keep your spine straight and focus your eyes on one spot to help you balance.

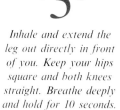

3

Inhale and extend the leg out directly in front of you. Keep your hips square and both knees straight. Breathe deeply and hold for 10 seconds.

4

Inhale and shift your weight to your heel. Do not bend the standing knee. Flex your foot harder, pull your stomach in, bend your elbows and stretch forward from the base of your spine, keeping your spine straight. Drop your forehead down to your knee and hold for as long as possible, breathing deeply. Repeat on the other side.

Standing Bow

This graceful exercise, called the Standing Bow because of the curve of the spine, will give you a sense of elation and power when you hold the pose as long as possible. The energy is continuously flowing in a circular pattern and as you increase the stretch your breathing pattern will quicken. Breathe deeply from the diaphragm to increase energy levels. This exercise will rejuvenate your spine and give you a sense of joy. Your circulation will be greatly improved and your whole body toned.

1

Stand up straight with your arms at your sides. Take your right leg behind you and hold the inner side of your foot. Straighten your elbow.

2

Take your left arm up close to your ear. Keep both shoulders down and look straight ahead. Breathe normally and steady your balance.

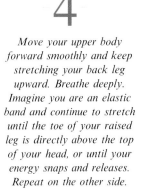

4

*Move your upper body
forward smoothly and keep
stretching your back leg
upward. Breathe deeply.
Imagine you are an elastic
band and continue to stretch
until the toe of your raised
leg is directly above the top
of your head, or until your
energy snaps and releases.
Repeat on the other side.*

3

*Inhale, lift the right leg
up from the hip as high
as possible and then
extend the left arm
forward. Breathing
normally, stretch in
opposite directions.*

Half Moon

This asana conveys harmony, balance, poise and power. It will give you a sense of achievement to flow into the final pose gracefully, without jerking. Before you begin the exercise, imagine yourself in the final position and feel as if you are a dancer as you move from one step to the next. The Half Moon also strengthens and tones the leg muscles and improves concentration.

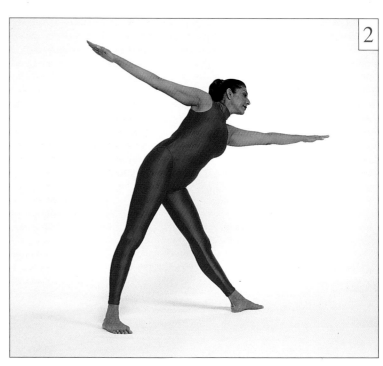

Stand in a wide second position with arms outstretched to the sides.

Tips

♦ *If the alignment of your spine and limbs are not perfect in Step 4, you will not be able to raise your leg with ease.*

♦ *Looking over your shoulder in the final position is an ultimate challenge because it means you are in perfect balance. As you turn your head, do not jerk or move the body. Look immediately to one point and steady your gaze – otherwise you will tumble down.*

♦ *Challenge yourself by trying to hold the final position for longer each time.*

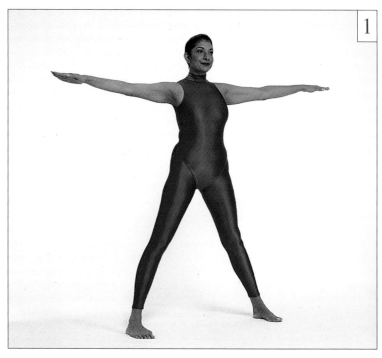

Breathing normally, turn your left foot to the left at a 90° angle. Make sure your left heel is in a direct line with the instep of the right foot. Stretch from the base of the spine to the left side.

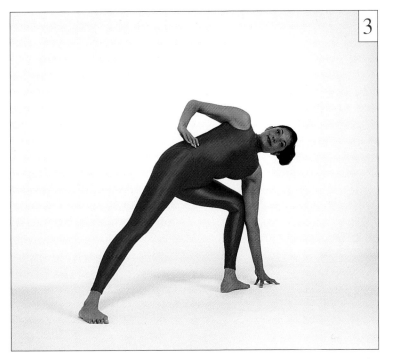

Bend your left knee, take your right hand to your waist and place your left hand on the floor. Look straight ahead and steady your balance. Breathe normally.

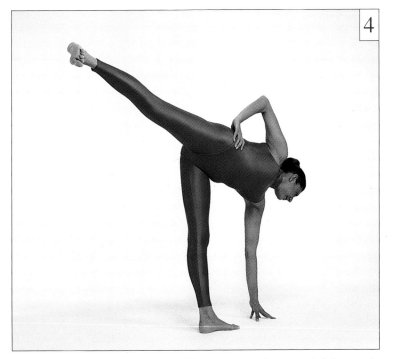

Focus on one spot on the floor. Inhale as you straighten your left knee and raise your right leg off the floor. Breathing normally, hold as long as possible; look over your right shoulder if you can. Repeat on the other side.

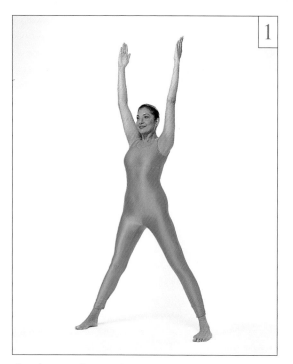

Stand in a wide second position with your feet 1m (3ft) apart. Throw your arms up with your elbows straight and palms facing each other.

Lunge with Balance

This exercise strengthens and tones all the muscles of the legs, stomach and arms. It builds stamina and suppleness of the spine. The position of the back stimulates the heartbeat and, with the increased oxygen pumped to the lungs, rejuvenates and energizes the entire body. The aim is to increase the mind control over the body while focusing attention and concentration on the physical. It needs tremendous skill to master this exercise, so do not become discouraged if it takes some time to learn. When you are in this pose it gives you a sense of harmony, balance, poise and power. It is especially recommended for runners and dancers as it brings vigor, agility and good carriage.

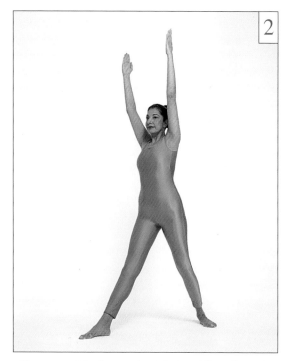

Turn your right foot to the right in a 90° angle to the left foot. Make sure the right heel is in line with the instep of the left foot. Breathe normally.

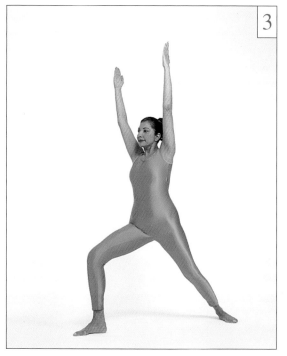

Lunge with your right leg and create a straight line from the back of the knee to the heel. You might need to adjust your left leg by taking it back further.

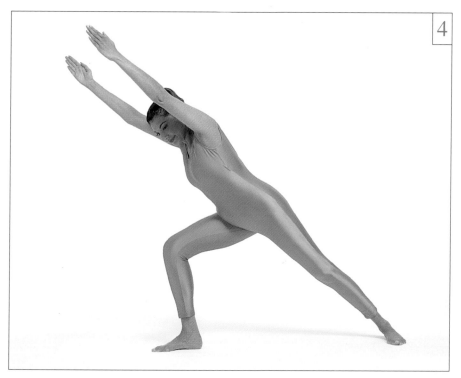

Take your body forward from the lower back so that your spine, arms and left leg are in an exact straight line. Focus your gaze on one spot on the floor. Inhale and exhale deeply.

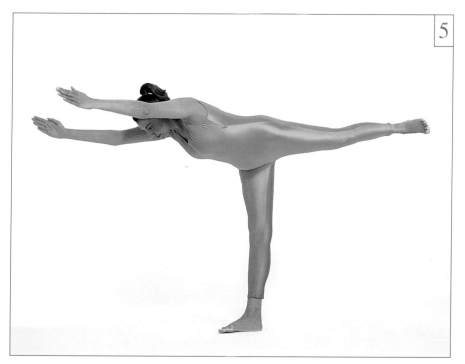

Inhale as you move your body forward and lift your left leg behind you. Flex the foot and try to keep parallel to the floor. Breathe deeply and hold as long as possible. Repeat on the other side.

Lunge with Back Twist

This, a variation of the previous exercise, calls for skill and a lot of determination. Pay special attention to the exact positioning of limbs, hands and feet. This is a powerful stretch, combining intense concentration with balance, suppleness, strength and stamina. Not only does it invigorate the internal organs, its deep twist releases toxins. If you feel sick and weak when you first begin this pose it means that your body is working to purify your system. Do not attempt Steps 4–7 until you have perfected Step 3.

1

Begin the pose as in Step 1 of previous exercise but with the arms outstretched to the sides. Change your foot positions as instructed in Step 2 of previous exercise and lunge to the right but do not twist the torso. Breathe normally.

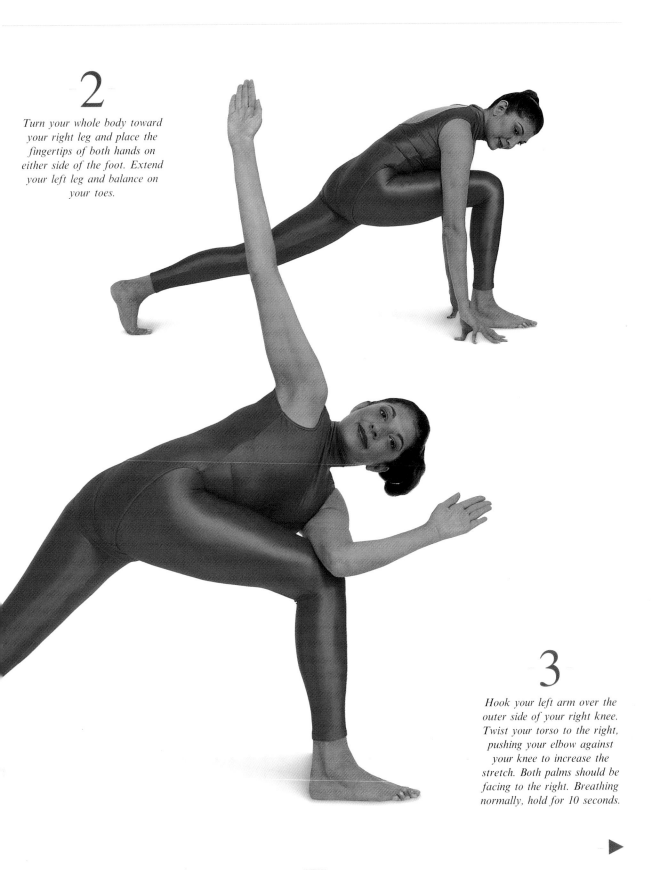

2

Turn your whole body toward your right leg and place the fingertips of both hands on either side of the foot. Extend your left leg and balance on your toes.

3

Hook your left arm over the outer side of your right knee. Twist your torso to the right, pushing your elbow against your knee to increase the stretch. Both palms should be facing to the right. Breathing normally, hold for 10 seconds.

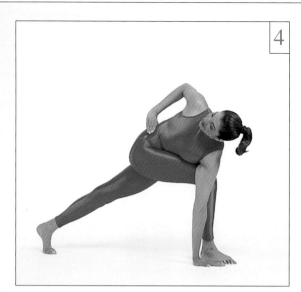

4

Place your left hand on the floor directly in line with your right foot. Place your right hand on your waist.

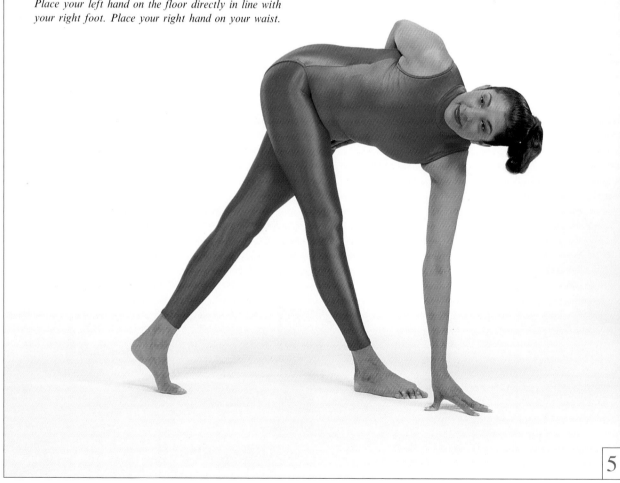

5

Straighten your right leg and shift your weight to your right foot in preparation for the next step.

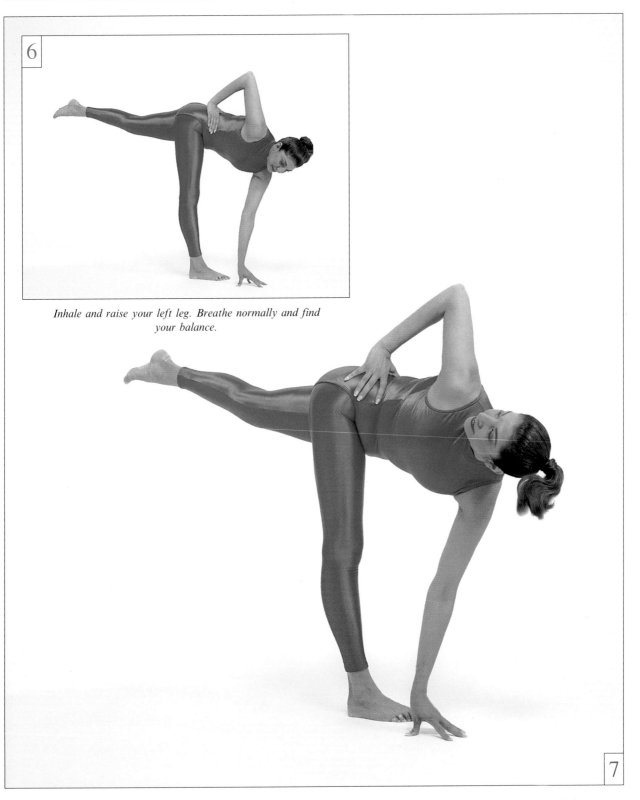

Inhale and raise your left leg. Breathe normally and find your balance.

When you are totally balanced, look over your right shoulder and increase the twist. Breathe normally and hold for as long as possible. Repeat on the other side.

Ultimate Twist

These two twists are classic positions to increase circulation in the spine and the abdominal organs, especially the liver and spleen. Twists cleanse and purify the system and are essential to the digestive system. Elimination is regulated, the kidneys are toned, and the blood circulation releases toxins that build up in the internal organs. When you are practicing twists you will find that every time you begin the pose it will be a different experience. As the flexibility of your spine increases you will be able to twist even further. Sluggishness will be replaced by higher energy levels and you will experience a feeling of youthfulness.

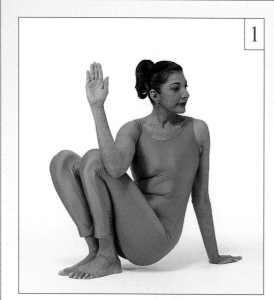

Sit with knees together and feet flat on the ground. Place your right elbow on the outside of your left knee and put your left hand on the floor in the opposite direction to your feet. Push against your knee and look over your left shoulder. Keeping your chin level and breathing normally, continue to stretch around. Hold for as long as you can. Repeat on the other side.

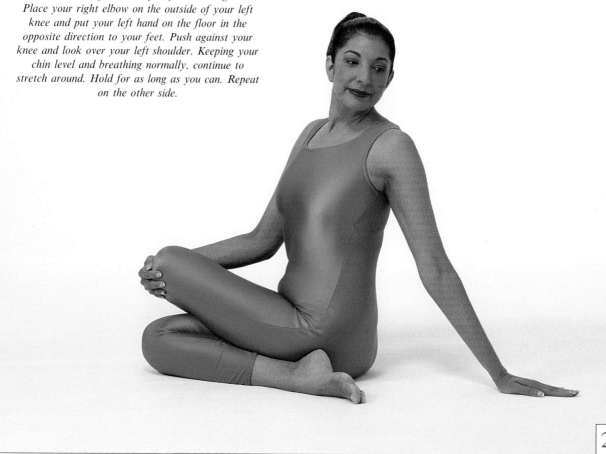

Sit with left leg over right leg. Take your right hand to the left knee and twist, looking as far over your left shoulder as possible. Place your left hand on the floor in line with your left leg. Breathe normally and continue to twist. Repeat on the other side.

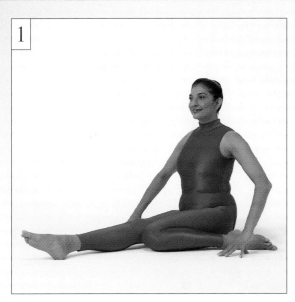

Sit with both legs extended in front. Bend your left knee and bring your heel to your hip. Place your fingertips on the floor on either side of your body. Breathe normally.

Leg Pull

The Leg Pull increases the flexibility of the hamstrings and tones muscle in the knees and legs. It also tones the spine and massages the abdominal wall; blood flows around the navel and rejuvenates the genital organs. Never lift the knee that is resting on the floor – if there is too much of a pull on the kneecap do not extend your chin all the way to your knee.

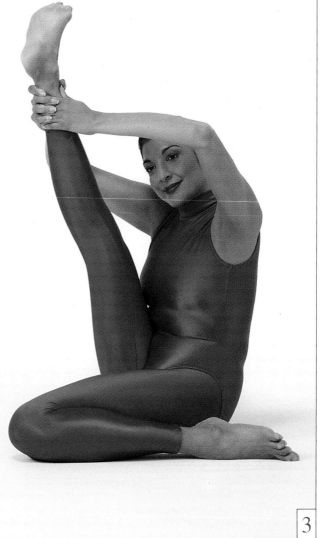

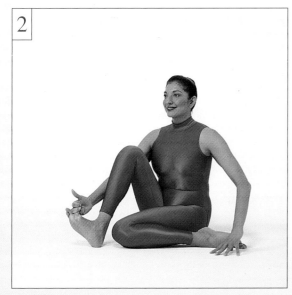

Bend your right knee and clasp your first two fingers around your big toe. Flex your thumb and right foot and prepare for the stretch.

Keeping your spine straight, inhale and stretch the leg up in front of you. Hold your ankle and pull your leg towards you. Breathing slowly and evenly, hold for 20 seconds. If you can, place your chin and forehead to the leg. Repeat on the other side.

Total Stretch

This stretch is very controversial – some people find it excruciating, while others feel it to be the most marvelous of all the classic stretches. The truth is that the more flexible you are the easier the pose. It stretches every muscle in the thighs, knees and ankles, as well the entire spine. If you feel any pain in your back, place a pillow under the small of the back and open your chest. If you feel your knees are strained place a small pillow under the back of your knees. The most important thing to remember is to relax in the position. Breathe deeply and evenly and feel the chest and hips open.

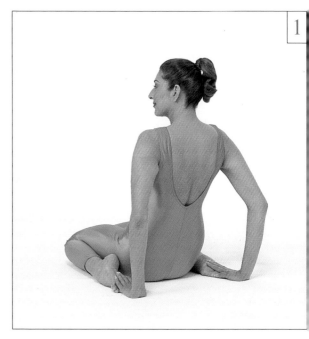

Sit upright and bring your knees together. Spread your feet and rest them either side of your hips, with your buttocks on the floor. Place your palms facing forward on your feet.

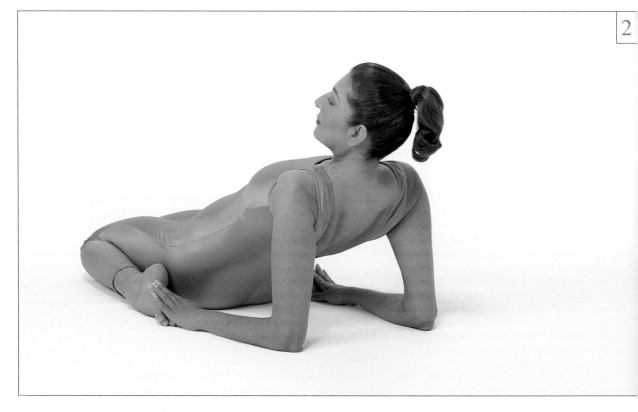

Drop your body back down, taking your weight on your elbows, and feel the stretch in your legs and abdomen.

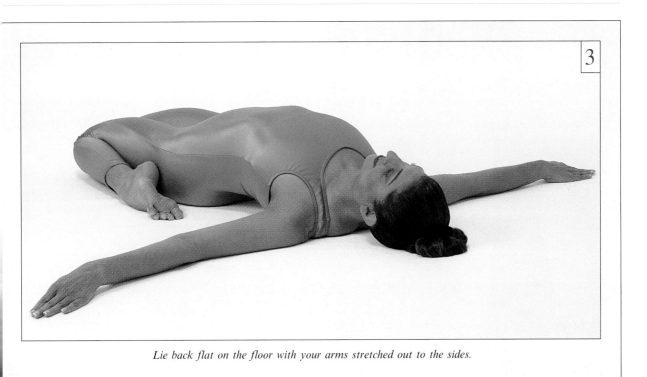

Lie back flat on the floor with your arms stretched out to the sides.

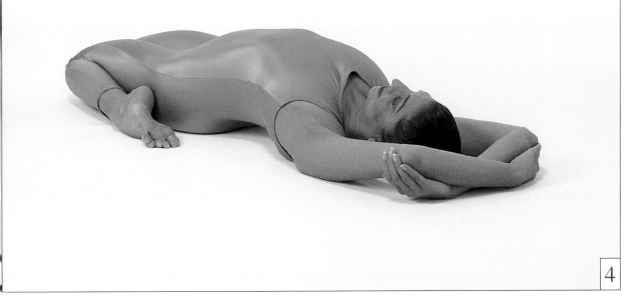

Clasp your elbows. Continue to breathe deeply and relax the entire body and mind. Try to hold this position for as long as possible – with practise you will be able to sustain it for 10–15 minutes.

Shoulder Stand

This is one of the most important asanas in classical yoga. Its benefits are many, the most important being that it stimulates and regulates the thyroid and parathyroid glands. Because of the chinlock, menstrual cycles regularize and weight remains stable. Healthy blood flows through the neck and chest, curing respiratory ailments and preventing sinus troubles and colds. Daily practice of this exercise cleanses the bowels and eliminates toxins.

2

Exhale and raise your legs to a 90° angle with your body, pointing your toes.

3

Inhale and take your legs over your head into the Plough position. Inhale and exhale.

1

Lie flat on the floor with your arms at your sides. Inhale and bring your knees into your chest.

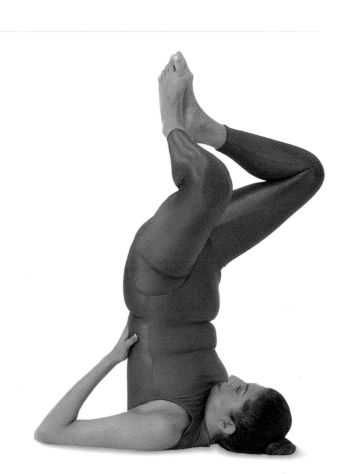

5

Bend your knees and
bring the soles of
your feet together.

4

Inhale and raise both legs as
high as possible – the aim is to
straighten the spine completely.
Lock your chin, point your toes
and place your hands in the
small of your back to support
your spine. Hold for 30 seconds,
breathing normally.

▶

6

Straighten both legs behind you. Tuck your toes under, and breathing deeply, walk both feet to the right side of your head.

7

Drop both knees as close to your right ear as possible. Straighten both legs and walk your feet to the left, then drop your knees as close to your left ear as possible.

8

Bring both legs directly behind your head. Point your toes. Inhale and raise both legs directly parallel to the floor. Breathe normally.

9

Bend both knees and change the position of your hands, so your thumbs are on your tail bone and your fingers are on your waist.

10

Straighten your spine and split your legs, creating a 90° angle with your left leg. Repeat on the other side.

▶

11

Return to the classic Shoulder Stand and hold for 10 seconds.

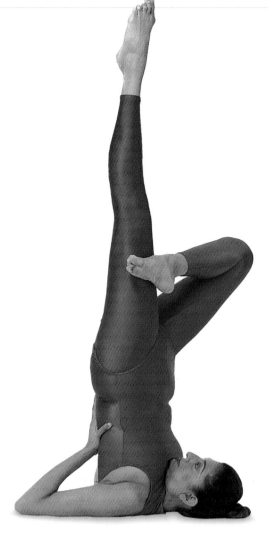

12

Bend your right leg and place the outer side of your foot against your left thigh just above your knee.

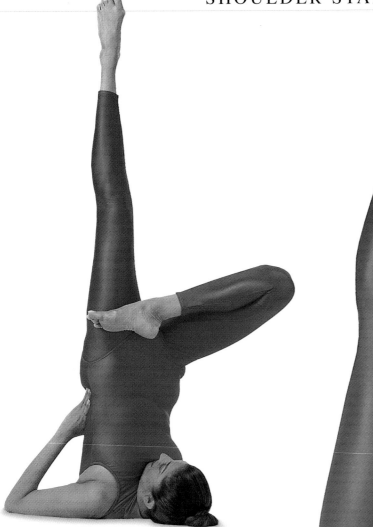

14

Return to the classic Shoulder Stand and hold for 10 seconds.

13

Bring your right heel toward your left hipbone. Push the knee back so it is square with the left hip. Return to Step 11 and repeat 12 and 13 on the other side.

17

Twist the entire spine to the left. Return to center and rotate to the right side.

16

Push both hips back so they are square.

15

Begin the lotus position. Bend your right leg and with your left hand pull the right foot in as close to the left hipbone as possible. Repeat on the other side.

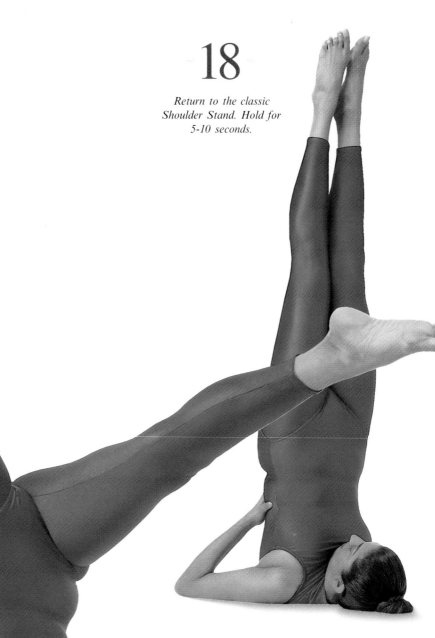

18

*Return to the classic
Shoulder Stand. Hold for
5-10 seconds.*

19

*Repeat Step 10 but extend the right leg.
Point the toes of both feet.*

▶

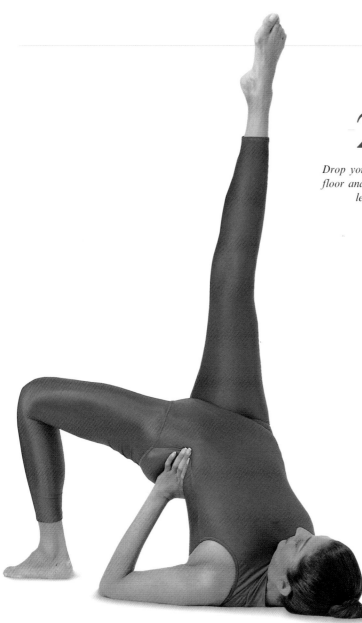

20

Drop your left foot to the floor and point your right leg upward.

21

Bend your right knee and place both feet on the floor. Raise your hips as high as possible. Breathe normally.

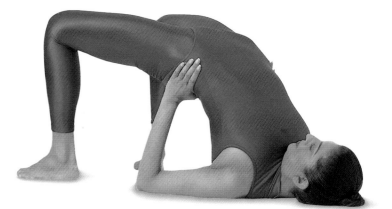

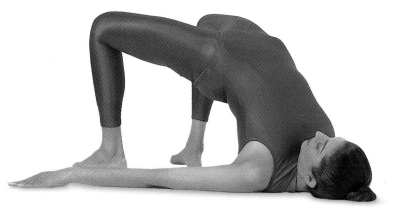

22

Take your hands down to the floor and continue to raise your hips.

23

Exhale slowly and, working from the top of the spine, slowly lower one vertebra at a time until your spine is completely flat on the floor.

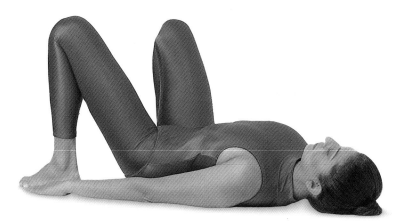

24

Relax your legs down to the floor and release your spine into the deep relaxation or Dead Man's pose. Relax for 5 minutes.

Head Stand

1

Kneel on the floor. Interlock your fingers, cross your thumbs and place your arms on the floor. Breathe normally.

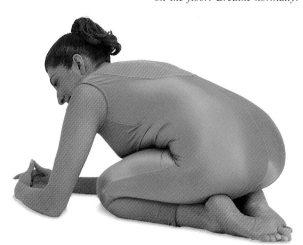

The Head Stand is called the king of all yoga asanas because it stimulates the pituitary and pineal glands. It is the gland that controls the brain, the seat of all wisdom, intelligence, discrimination and reasoning power. Without a healthy brain you cannot function. The inverted position of the Head Stand allows the blood to flow freely to the brain and feeds the brain cells with fresh oxygen. It gives you clarity of mind and wards off senility as you age. The brain also controls the entire nervous system and during the practice of the Head Stand all the nerves and cells are being rejuvenated. Health and vitality are restored and when you practice it on a regular basis you will develop the body, discipline the mind and broaden the spirit.

2

Making sure your elbows are directly under your shoulder blades, place the top of your head down on the floor just in front of your hands.

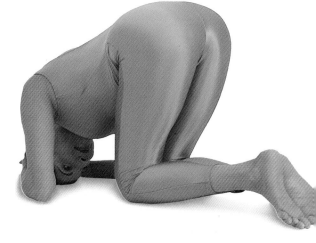

3

Tuck your toes under and spring up onto your toes with your legs straight. Walk your feet toward your head until your spine is straight.

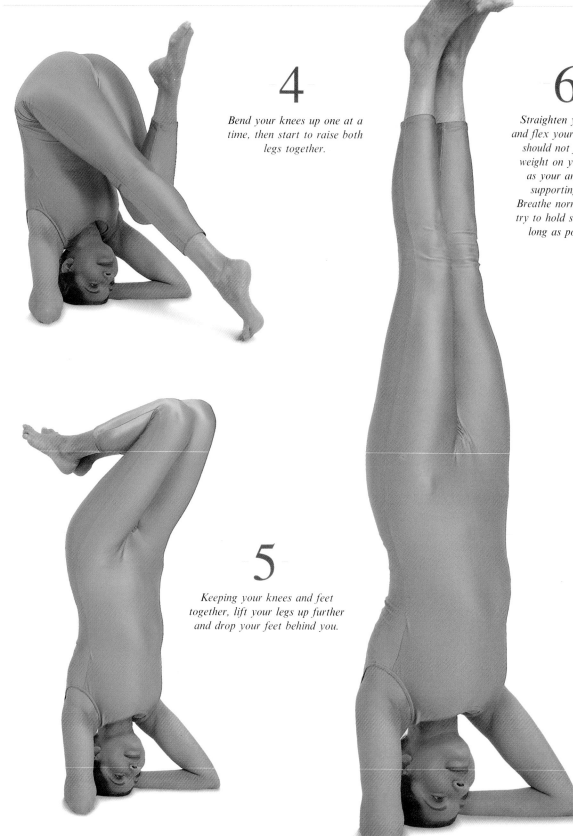

4

Bend your knees up one at a time, then start to raise both legs together.

6

Straighten your legs and flex your toes. You should not feel any weight on your head as your arms are supporting you. Breathe normally and try to hold still for as long as possible.

5

Keeping your knees and feet together, lift your legs up further and drop your feet behind you.

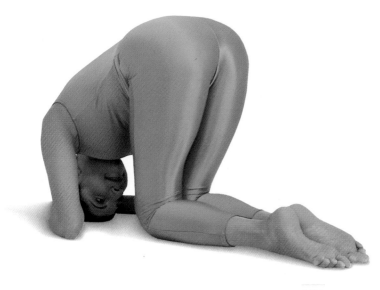

7

Open your legs to second position, keeping your feet flexed. Hold for 10 seconds.

8

Bend your knees at a right angle.

9

Slowly bring your knees forward, curving your spine, and return to the floor. Stay in this position for 10 seconds. If you come up suddenly you will feel dizzy.

Uddiyana

In Sanskrit, 'Uddiyana' means 'flying up'. In this exercise the air is drawn up from the lower abdomen and moves under the ribcage toward the head. This movement tones the abdominal organs, increases the gastric juices and eliminates toxins in the digestive tract. It is a wonderful way to exercise the muscles of the stomach, thereby making it flatter.

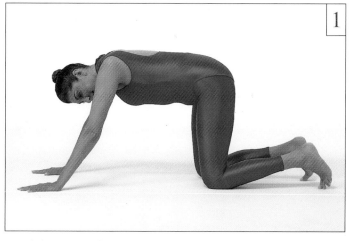

Kneel down on all fours. Keep your spine straight and place your hands and feet in a direct line. Inhale through your nose and exhale through your mouth until all the breath is out of your lungs.

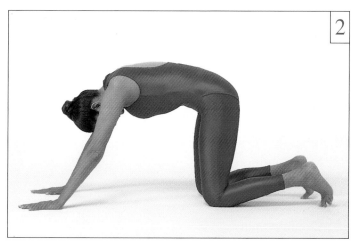

Pull the stomach muscles up and curve your spine slightly. Without taking a breath, contract and release the muscles to massage the internal organs. When you tire, inhale and exhale normally for a few breaths. Repeat the whole exercise up to 20 times.

Acknowledgements

Executive Editor	Sian Facer
Art Director	Keith Martin
Design	Martin Topping
Editors	Jane McIntosh
	Mary Lambert
	Diana Vowles
Production	Melanie Frantz
	Candida Lane
Photography	John Adriaan
Hair and Make-up	Leslie Sayles
Director of Photography	Jon Acevski